Ultimate Abs

The Definitive Guide
to Developing a Chiseled Six-Pack

Ultimate Abs

The Definitive Guide to Developing a Chiseled Six-Pack

Gareth Sapstead

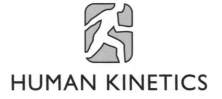

HUMAN KINETICS

Library of Congress Cataloging-in-Publication Data

Names: Sapstead, Gareth, author.
Title: Ultimate abs : the definitive guide to developing a chiseled six-pack / Gareth Sapstead.
Description: Champaign, IL : Human Kinetics, 2022. | Includes bibliographical references.
Identifiers: LCCN 2020057354 (print) | LCCN 2020057355 (ebook) | ISBN 9781718201392 (paperback) | ISBN 9781718201408 (epub) | ISBN 9781718201415 (pdf)
Subjects: LCSH: Abdominal exercises. | Abdomen--Muscles.
Classification: LCC GV508 .S27 2022 (print) | LCC GV508 (ebook) | DDC 613.7/1886--dc23
LC record available at https://lccn.loc.gov/2020057354
LC ebook record available at https://lccn.loc.gov/2020057355

ISBN: 978-1-7182-0139-2 (print)

Acquisitions Editor: Michael Mejia; **Developmental Editor:** Amy Stahl; **Copyeditor:** Annette Pierce; **Proofreader:** Pamela S. Johnson; **Permissions Manager:** Martha Gullo; **Graphic Designer:** Dawn Sills; **Cover Designer:** Keri Evans; **Cover Design Specialist:** Susan Rothermel Allen; **Photograph (cover):** vuk8691 / iStock/Getty Images; **Photographs (interior):** © Human Kinetics; **Photo Production Specialist:** Amy M. Rose; **Photo Production Manager:** Jason Allen; **Senior Art Manager:** Kelly Hendren; **Illustrations:** © Human Kinetics; **Printer:** Sheridan Books

We thank KineticFitness in Nottingham, England, for assistance in providing the location for the photo shoot for this book.

Human Kinetics books are available at special discounts for bulk purchase. Special editions or book excerpts can also be created to specification. For details, contact the Special Sales Manager at Human Kinetics.

Printed in the United States of America   10 9 8 7 6 5 4 3 2 1

The paper in this book is certified under a sustainable forestry program.

Human Kinetics
1607 N. Market Street
Champaign, IL 61820
USA

United States and International
Website: **US.HumanKinetics.com**
Email: info@hkusa.com
Phone: 1-800-747-4457

Canada
Website: **Canada.HumanKinetics.com**
Email: info@hkcanada.com

E8236

Tell us what you think!
Human Kinetics would love to hear what we can do to improve the customer experience. Use this QR code to take our brief survey.

This book is dedicated to my family and friends. You all know who you are, and without your love and support, I wouldn't be the person you see today. Above all, to Alex and Ozzie for walking through this awesome life with me.

Contents

PART III   THE PROGRAMS   205

Exercise Finder

Exercise	Difficulty level	Page number
Chapter 4 Using Cardio as a Tool		
Shuttle Run	N/A	49
Agility Run	N/A	50
Basic Sled Push	N/A	51
Battle Ropes	N/A	52
Basic Farmer's Carry	N/A	53
Rowing Machine	N/A	54
Treadmill	N/A	55
Cycling, Spinning, and Air Bike	N/A	56
Elliptical Trainer	N/A	57
Boxing Bag	N/A	58
Chapter 7 Captain Crunch: Targeting Your Spine		
Basic Abdominal Crunch	Foundational	76
Stability Ball Crunch	Intermediate	78
Cable Stability Ball Crunch	Advanced	79
Hamstring-Activated Sit-Up	Advanced	80
Hamstring-Activated Stability Ball Crunch	Advanced	81
Lying Banded Crunch	Intermediate	82
Lying Banded Elbows to Knees	Intermediate	83
Standing Heavy-Band Crunch	Foundational	84
Kneeling Cable Crunch	Foundational	85
Standing Cable Crunch	Intermediate	86
Landmine Crunch	Advanced	87
Crunch With a Lat Pull-Down Machine	Advanced	88
Incline Eccentric Cable Crunch	Hardcore	89
Abdominal V-Up	Intermediate	90
Ab Mat Crunch	Foundational	91
Dumbbell Serratus Crunch	Intermediate	92
Dead-Bug Crunch	Intermediate	93
High-Pulley Cable Crunch on Stability Ball	Advanced	94
Low-Pulley Cable Crunch	Intermediate	95
Sicilian Crunch	Advanced	96
Overhead Medicine Ball Slam	Intermediate	97
Plate Over Knee Crunch	Intermediate	98
Heavy Battle Rope Slam	Intermediate	99
Ab Wheel Rollout With Flexion	Intermediate	100
Seated Ab Cable Crunch	Intermediate	101

(continued)

(continued)

Preface

You want six-pack abs. You've probably realized by now that it takes far more than just endless crunches to achieve your goal. You're finally ready to approach your mission with a more clearly designed system of training and exercises to guarantee your success. *Ultimate Abs: The Definitive Guide to Building a Chiseled Six-Pack* makes no secret of what this system is. From the first to last page, there's one aim: to provide the tools and exercises you need in order to build a chiseled six-pack—and then some.

Your abs, you see, contribute much more than just looking good on the beach or when wearing a tight T-shirt. As a collective, your abdominal muscles form one of the most important muscle groups. A well-conditioned midsection will improve your posture, manage back pain, and make you a better athlete. Using an intelligent approach to training and exercise selection, *Ultimate Abs* is a book for anyone and everyone who wants to look, feel, and perform better.

For some time now, the focus within common media has been on the concept of core strength training. Although stabilization exercises are included, *Ultimate Abs* is an unapologetic guide to developing chiseled six-pack abs; looks are the priority. Put simply, by focusing on this specific objective, *Ultimate Abs* will help you achieve your goals faster.

Chapter 1 explores some of the misconceptions surrounding ab training and reveals the most effective way to develop a six-pack. While common practice is to perform endless repetitions of inferior exercises, I aim to redefine your approach to effective abdominal training. I also condense the science to basic and practical information that applies to all aspects of training.

Chapter 2 takes a dive into spine and abdominal anatomy. Understanding basic anatomical principles will allow you to better select exercises from later in the book. This in turn will allow you to train with more precision and targeted results. In particular, the chapter discusses the concept of spinal flexion, which is the act of bending your spine forward. Because spinal flexion has long been considered contraindicated for even the healthiest people, chapter 2 addresses the question once and for all: Is spinal flexion bad?

Chapter 3 clearly defines what abdominal training is and what differentiates it from more core-centric training. Core training largely focuses on exercises that strengthen and stabilize the lumbo–pelvic–hip complex (i.e., the combined regions of the lower part of your spine, pelvis, and hips). It's an integrated approach that emphasizes the function of your midsection over that of its looks. Building on concepts already learned in chapters 1 and 2, chapter 3 will show you what types of exercise are the most important for a chiseled six-pack.

Cardiovascular conditioning might help you burn unwanted body fat but should be seen as merely a secondary tool. It's the side dish to your entree. Countless hours on a treadmill will not develop a cut and strong-looking midsection. If body fat covers your hard-earned six-pack muscles, it's important to achieve a caloric deficit in order to unveil it. Chapter 4 covers how to effectively use cardiovascular exercise to carve out your six-pack only if and when it's required. Chapter 5 then shows you exactly how to track your body changes accurately.

Chapter 6, Selecting the Best Exercises, shows you how to identify exercises that will work for you and your body. While cookie-cutter abdominal routines are common, this chapter will teach you to identify what's right for you. This will make your workout time more productive and result in more long-term success with less injury. *Ultimate Abs* is about maximizing abdominal training efficiency and using tools and learning concepts that will provide a lifetime of results.

Chapters 7 through 10 are the meat and potatoes of this book. This comprehensive overview of more than 100 of the best exercises to help you achieve a chiseled six-pack is what differentiates this book from all others. Each exercise was carefully selected from a list of thousands as being the most effective. Each chapter outlines the best exercises for each area of your core: spine, upper abs, stubborn lower abs, and obliques. You'll understand exactly why and how each exercise works.

Although you'll want to try every exercise in this book—there are unique and exciting variations—first understanding how an exercise works will keep you on the straight and narrow path to six-pack success. Chapter 10, Planks and Other "Anti" Movements, provides options when total back health and performance are a priority.

Building muscle strength and six-pack abs is the clear subject of this book, but this should not be at the expense of your overall health and pain-free performance. Chapter 11 provides the top six exercises to complement your six-pack workouts. The chapter includes the high-value exercises that will strengthen your glutes, lower back, and other key areas.

The programs in chapters 12 through 14 combine some of the most beneficial exercises that were described in detail in prior chapters. There are nine programs, which cover every scenario and level. Whether you want to work out using just your own body weight from home with little equipment or work out at a gym, there's a routine with your name on it.

Finally, chapter 15 builds from everything you have learned and takes things up a level by teaching you how to develop and structure your own program. You'll gain a deeper understanding of how to pick the best exercises for your body and goals, the principle of specificity, important programming concepts, and even how to work around common injuries. This section is based on both scientific principles and tens of thousands of hours of real-world coaching practice.

Ultimate Abs provides highly valuable and useable information in each chapter, backed up by scientifically founded principles. Each chapter can be used as a stand-alone resource or pieced together to form the definitive guide to six-pack abs. If you're a fitness professional you'll appreciate the depth with which each exercise is presented, and everyone from beginner to advanced will be inspired to use and share it. If you want to build a chiseled six-pack and get the most out of your training, dive right in, and start learning how.

Introduction

It wouldn't take a genius to figure out what you want most. You've just picked up and opened a book that has the title *Ultimate Abs*. Chances are pretty high then, that what you want are big pecs and bulging biceps. Just kidding! Sure, you probably want those too, but you've not picked up a book on training those body parts have you?

The desire for six-pack abs runs through the veins of every man. From depictions of ancient gladiators to the front cover of just about every fitness magazine you see today, it's the one body part we desire chiseled above all others. Yet it is a goal few of us ever achieve.

A chiseled midsection is the ultimate show of strength, athleticism, and virility throughout many cultures. Attaining one demonstrates discipline and the ability to push yourself in areas of your life where many won't. Having low levels of body fat is one thing, but to build abs that not only look good but also perform well are the envy of every man.

Years of spinning your wheels in the dirt and sweating over endless ab exercises have probably made you frustrated. Putting the time and effort in with very little return would do that to anyone. Instead of leaving sweat angels on floors, you could have spent that time doing other things—playing and watching sports or playing video games; you get the picture. Or you could have spent time with family, of course.

Better yet, it's time you could have spent on a more efficient path—one that guarantees six-pack abs at the end of it. This book *is* that path and will allow you to identify, once and for all, the best methods and exercises to achieve six-pack success. This is a book for all men who want those "damn, I look good" kind of results and men frustrated and bored with common and ineffective ab and core routines.

From the get-go, this book will throw at you the best advice that not only will benefit you right now, but also will become a valuable resource you'll want to dive in to time and time again. You'll get the most from this book by reading it from front to back cover, but equally, you'll be able to open to any page and find something of interest. It is a user-friendly and highly practical guide to building a chiseled six-pack and one that will inspire both your immediate and long-term progress.

Initially, I'll outline what it truly takes and the process behind getting and maintaining chiseled six-pack abs. Whether you struggle with stubborn abdominal fat or can't etch abs deep enough, this book will condense the science into real-world advice that'll help you overcome any obstacle. As someone who suffered from "paralysis by overanalysis" in the past, I understand how making this information as concise as possible will allow you to follow the clearest path to success.

Sure, feel free to read as many exercise science textbooks as you can get your hands on. This publisher leads the way in those. However, if you want to truly end the frustration and eliminate the program hopping that has held you back in the past, let this book be your only guide. Everything you need to know is in front of you, and what you don't has been purposely left out.

Here's a useful analogy to consider. Let's say that you wake up and decide to take a quick run down to your local coffee shop before work. Maybe you've run out of coffee at home and desperately need caffeine to function. Once you get there, you notice that because it's prime time, there's a queue. No big deal, you've accounted for the wait. But then you notice the pastry counter as well as the fancy new iced tea they're offering. So you order one of those and a cinnamon bun. You get home and realize you don't have the coffee you went out for. The iced tea tastes bad and like it's from a packet mix, and the cinnamon bun is the last of yesterday's batch. The rest of your morning is ruined. Heck, you might as well make it the entire day!

The point is you went out for coffee. You put in the time and effort to get one but were persuaded to buy shiny and sugary things instead. Next time you go out for a coffee, make sure you come back with one. If it's six-pack abs you want, then train for six-pack abs.

Now here comes the exciting bit. After you have context and an understanding of ab-building principles and common myths, you also have more than 100 exercises to start applying to your own training. Now, maybe 100-plus exercises doesn't sound that impressive to you. But consider that by the end of reading this book, you'll know more about each of these exercises than you could ever imagine. You'll understand exactly why and how to use each exercise as well as understand the more complex exercise mechanics that are condensed into their simplest and most understandable form—information you can actually apply.

In the process of learning about each exercise, you'll also discover why you've sacrificed on progress in the past. A wise man once told me, "The more you know about training and programming, the less exercise options there are." Following that principle, I have included only the exercises that work and deserve your time and attention.

You'll likely notice that what you have been led to believe about core training has in fact been holding you back from your ultimate goal. While having a strong core is important—we'll discuss this in chapter 3—it's not the most efficient path to six-pack abs. It's going out to get a coffee and instead coming back with an iced tea.

Throughout common media, *core* has largely been used as a marketing term. Because of this, it has somewhat lost its true meaning and caused confusion—confusion that has caused many to fall off the correct path. This book aims to strap you up to rocket-boosted skates and put you back on it. There are no ineffective routines and exercises. There is no more talk of core. That's important, of course, but visible abs are *the* goal. No more gimmicks. From here on out, you'll hear only about the things that will work. There'll be no apologies for the barriers this book will help you break through. Enjoy the journey.

Acknowledgments

First and foremost, I'd like to thank the entire Human Kinetics family—with a special thanks to Mike Mejia and Amy Stahl for allowing my vision of this book to become a reality. I want to thank everyone who ever gave me an opportunity to share my ideas to the world, especially Chris Shugart and the team at T-Nation.

I've had a lot of mentors and friends in the fitness industry and have been influenced by far too many to name. While postgraduate study and college professors taught me critical thinking, others with skin in the game taught me to think outside of the box. Years of working with my awesome clients and athletes have also shaped my training philosophy immensely. No problem is too complex to solve, and no amount of stubborn ab fat is too hard to chisel! This mix of evidence-based and real-world experience is one that I hope you'll recognize as a theme throughout this book.

Finally, thanks to the people I'm closest to daily and frequently bounce ideas off in both fitness and business. This group includes my brother and fellow fitness pro, Ryan Sapstead, for never sugarcoating it and always being my fiercest critic. And to superfriend Chris Stankiewicz—I recall a time some years back, while working on a book we coauthored for another publisher, when we daydreamed that one day it would instead be for Human Kinetics. My passion for this book is something only Chris knows.

I hope this book serves you for a lifetime of health, fitness, and rock-hard abs.

The Scientific Approach to Ab Training

Part I teaches the scientific principles that underpin effective ab training. This section takes complex subjects and condenses them into information that you can apply. Understanding the training philosophy outlined in this book and learning these core concepts will give you the solid foundation of knowledge on which to build your ab training. Taking this scientific approach to ab training allows you to understand why some exercises and techniques work while others don't and why certain exercises are included in part II while others didn't make the cut.

We begin part I with a journey through the basic ab-building principles and concepts that translate into the training of your entire physique. You'll learn the different muscle actions and how to use them, the effect of training muscles at different lengths, the science behind sets and repetitions (and which reps *really* are best for your abs), and what it takes for your abs to grow and become more deeply etched.

Next, in chapter 2, we'll explore spinal and abdominal anatomy. You'll learn the muscles that compose the abdominal wall and obliques and learn which exercises most effectively train them. This leads us into important questions: Will abdominal crunches hurt my back and is spinal flexion really that bad?

The terms *core training* and *ab training* are frequently used interchangeably. In chapter 3, you'll learn why this often creates confusion and the real difference between core and ab training. After reading this chapter, you'll know how to avoid some of the key mistakes many people make in their pursuit of six-pack abs. You'll learn to narrow your goals and better identify the exercises that will help you achieve them. You'll also learn how to combine different types of exercises for the most impressive results.

It's frequently suggested that abs are built in the kitchen. In chapter 4, you'll find out why this just isn't the case. You'll also be taken through a lesson on energy balance and how cardiovascular exercise can play a role in losing stubborn abdominal fat. We also discuss nutrition and how it factors into energy balance. Chapter 4 culminates with a detailed description of the best cardio exercises for attaining six-pack abs. This is cardio you'll actually look forward to doing.

Finally, chapter 5 will show you how to track your six-pack progress. If you're not using one of these methods to track your progress, then you need to start right away. What you monitor, you can manage; if you are accurately monitoring changes to your physique, then you'll be better able to manage the transformation of your entire body. Every ounce of information in part I is integral to your successful use of the exercises (part II) and programs (part III). If you understand the "why" of exercise selection and how these influence your progress, then you'll enjoy the process a whole lot more.

Ab-Building Principles

The goal of this book is a practical one. Every piece of information is something you can take action on and implement within your own training plan. That being said, a basic understanding of the principles that underpin exercise selection and program design will help you better put them into action. We'll start with the basics.

RESISTANCE TRAINING

Whether you're picking up a barbell or pushing yourself up from the floor, you're exposing your muscles to some form of resistance, also known as resistance training. Every time you perform, say, a crunch off the floor, complex systems are working together. While you're doing this and concerned with training your abs, your body usually has other ideas.

As you're performing each crunch, your body is finding the most efficient way to get from point A (the floor) to point B (shoulders lifted off the floor). Your brain and neuromuscular system don't care that you're trying to work your abs. Your body is lazy, but it's lazy for a reason. *Lazy* is just another way to say that it's efficient. It will always take the easiest path and expend the least amount of energy possible.

Your abdominal muscles do not have eyes that can see the outside of your body. They don't know the difference between you crunching with a dumbbell or a brick in your hands. Your abs also don't have emotions. They don't care that you're working as hard as you possibly can to make them look better. Later, in part II we'll show you how to upgrade your exercises and overcome abdominal laziness to get better results.

Muscles contract and cause joints to flex and movements to take place. How they do this is explored further in chapter 2. Muscles feel changes in tension. They adapt according to the signals you give them, and that's why it's important to send them the right signals.

THE PRINCIPLE OF SPECIFICITY

Commonly termed the *SAID principle* (specific adaptation to imposed demands), in the context of exercise, it describes how the human body adapts to the demands placed on it. It states that specific stressors on the human body—whether mechanical, physiological, or neurological—cause a specific adaptation, usually in a way that will help your body better deal with that stressor in the future.

An ab workout is a stressor, and each repetition of every set creates a small amount of stress that your body recognizes. Using the SAID principle, we can clearly state that the adaptation you want most is to grow a chiseled set of abs. In other words, you want muscular hypertrophy to take place in your abdominal region. Muscular hypertrophy is discussed later in the chapter.

Building abs doesn't mean that your waist will get thicker—much like your biceps popping out of your sleeves. Instead, your abdominals grow by becoming more dense and developing deeply etched lines. So, as much as you may want toned abs, you are in fact trying to *grow* them. Dropping the layer of body fat covering them wouldn't be a waste of time either.

Sending your body the right signals for this to happen is key. During typical core training, most of the time you're sending your body the wrong signals because you're spending the majority of your time doing the wrong things. Muscle building mechanisms as they pertain to your entire body, as they do your abdominals, are discussed in more detail later in this chapter.

TYPES OF MUSCLE ACTION

Exercises don't cause muscles to contract. It's the muscles contracting that produces the action, and there are three main types of muscle action you should know: concentric, eccentric, and isometric. We'll discuss these extensively because certain exercises emphasize certain types of contractions, and each brings unique benefits.

Concentric Actions

Concentric actions are characterized by muscles producing tension when shortening. For example, as you perform an abdominal crunch, while lifting yourself off the floor, your rectus abdominis will concentrically contract to pull your ribs toward your pelvis, flexing your spine. Another example is a simple knee raise where the action of your hip flexors begins the movement of pulling your knees toward your chest.

Specific characteristics of concentric muscle actions are worth talking about here because the majority of resistance exercises involve a concentric action. Special methods can emphasize the concentric phase of an exercise, which offers unique benefits.

Concentric actions require more energy and produce greater levels of muscle activation and more metabolite accumulation than eccentric actions do (Dalton and Stokes 1991; Kraemer et al. 2006). Because of this, repeated concentric actions are responsible for the burn you feel during a high-repetition set of any exercise. That burning sensation is a result of and accompanied by an increase in lactate, positive hydrogen ions, and blood ammonia, among other things. This metabolic stress can lead to several downstream effects, including an increase in growth hormone (GH) and insulin-like growth factor (IGF-1). These can rev up your muscle-building and fat-burning potential.

To make the concentric phase of lifting as effective as possible, the focus should be on maximizing muscle tension. Picking the best exercises to achieve this is just one of the goals of this book. To maximize tension, you need to produce high levels of force.

In physics, force equals mass times acceleration ($F = m \times a$). If we understand this, then it's clear that in order to produce high levels of muscular force during the concentric phase, we must do one of two things. Either we must lift heavy weights slower or lift lighter weights more explosively. The laws of physics apply just the same whether you are heavy squatting or performing an exercise to target your abs. By emphasizing the concentric and deemphasizing the eccentric phase of an exercise, you can control muscle damage, reduce muscle soreness, and even train with a higher frequency. Part II covers exercise techniques and coaching cues to help you achieve this.

Eccentric Actions

During eccentric actions, your muscles produce tension when lengthening. In the example of an abdominal crunch, your muscles contract concentrically as you raise your shoulders off the floor. Then, as you lower, your abdominals contract eccentrically to control the movement.

Studies have shown that maximal strength can be 20 to 50 percent greater during eccentric contractions than during concentric muscle actions (Schoenfeld et al. 2017). The reasons for this aren't well understood, but a giant elastic muscle protein called *titin* is likely responsible. Titin acts as a form of scaffolding for some of the internal muscle structures, providing additional stiffness as muscles lengthen. This additional stiffness might explain why eccentric muscle actions produce greater levels of force but lower levels of overall muscle activation and fewer energy requirements.

Most common exercises include both a concentric and eccentric phase. To overload a muscle eccentrically, you must perform a longer-duration eccentric action or lift more weight than you can concentrically. On top of overall greater force production, capitalizing on other unique benefits of eccentric training can help with muscle development. These types of exercises produce high levels of mechanical tension and muscle damage, both of which are important for building muscle. Studies have shown that eccentric training leads to more muscle hypertrophy than concentric-based training does (De Souza-Teixeira and De Paz 2012; Schoenfeld et al. 2017).

Certain exercises and special methods can make the most of the unique benefits of eccentric training. These exercises are included in part II.

Isometric Actions

During isometric actions, the muscles produce tension without changing length or joint angle. For example, imagine performing an abdominal crunch and holding your position for a few seconds at the top of each repetition. This static position requires an isometric muscle action.

Isometric exercises can also be broken into what are commonly referred to as eccentric and concentric isometrics. Eccentric isometric exercises require you to hold resistance while fighting to keep it from pulling you down, sometimes all the way until you reach failure. An example of this would be using the bench press exercise and simply holding the bar at the top while resisting the downward movement. The basic plank exercise might also be considered a form of eccentric isometric as you fight gravity from dropping your hips towards the floor.

A concentric isometric exercise, on the other hand, requires you to apply a force directly against something that doesn't move. Imagine pressing against an immovable object as hard as you can when you reach the top of a crunch.

Emphasizing isometric muscle actions leads to significant and unique benefits. Theoretically, isometric training can create a large amount of mechanical tension and metabolic stress. These contribute to building work capacity, connective tissue health, strength, and muscle size (Oranchuk et al. 2019).

Very high levels of muscle activation and tension can be achieved during isometric exercises, so your abs have not likely benefitted from the low-load isometrics you've done in the past. And your basic body-weight planks are in need of a serious upgrade! The exercises in this book will show you how to load these exercises in the safest and most effective way.

COMPOUND VERSUS ISOLATION EXERCISES

Compound exercises are those that involve multiple joints and muscle groups. These exercises include your typical strength and bodybuilding movements such as squats, deadlifts, and bench presses. They should also form the larger part of your resistance training workouts because they offer the biggest payoff for the effort. Compound exercises activate the most muscle tissue and trigger key pathways involved in strength and muscle building. Compound exercises also offer the greatest carryover to sport and daily activities. As such, they're often described as being more functional.

Many coaches and trainers, especially those with a powerlifting background, focus their training on just a handful of compound lifts. They stress the importance of getting stronger in just these lifts without the need for many others. A lot can be said for this limited approach, but when training the abdominals specifically, a few things must be considered.

While it's true that compound exercises should provide the bulk of any good program, that does not mean that one should be limited to just a few of these exercises. Trying to fit yourself to an exercise rather than finding the right exercise to fit *you* is a sure path to cranky joints and injuries—not to mention the lack of progress you'd experience from such an approach. Compound exercises should form a key component within your overall training program, but find those that fit your unique body structure and history. This is the same whether you're selecting a squat variation or an exercise to work your abdominals. Later we'll cover how to select exercises to suit your unique body type, exercise history, and goals.

The second point to consider is that performing only big compound exercises is not enough to develop a strong core and six-pack abs. While using compound exercises progressively over time will indeed help, isolation exercises are often needed to target that area. That's especially true when referring to the more superficial abdominal muscles. For example, external oblique and rectus abdominis muscle activation is moderate at best during the back squat and does not appear to increase as the load gets heavier (Aspe and Swinton 2014).

Isolation exercises are movements that involve a single joint and focus on individual muscles. Because this book focuses on a small group of muscles, you'll find many exercises that fall under this category.

Since the rising popularity of more functional and core-based training approaches, the use of isolation exercises has largely been left to the bodybuilding community. These exercises are used to work isolated muscle groups and activate as much muscle tissue in that targeted area as possible. This approach can be compared to that of a sculptor spending time chiseling the areas of a statue that warrant perfecting. It would be smart to apply the same strategy to your own body.

Exercises that focus on the core involve compound movements. Multiple joints and muscle groups are involved, working more than just your abdominals. On the other hand, developing your more visible abdominal muscles requires focus and precision. In any training plan, there is a place for both strategies, and differences in strategies will be covered further in chapter 3.

MUSCLE-BUILDING MECHANISMS

Muscular hypertrophy is an increase in size of skeletal muscle through a growth in size of its component cells. It can be thought of as a thickening of muscle fibers. If you want to build muscle and chisel your abs, you should know the basic science behind it. This will help you understand and apply the exercises presented in part II. It will also help direct your entire approach to resistance training.

Two types of hypertrophy contribute to larger muscles: sarcoplasmic and myofibrillar hypertrophy. Sarcoplasmic hypertrophy is the increase in the size of the noncontractile components within the muscle, the fluid within the muscle. It is sometimes referred to as *nonfunctional* hypertrophy because it doesn't result in a muscle's ability to produce more force. If you've ever wondered why a person can look much stronger than he actually is, it's likely that his training results in greater sarcoplasmic hypertrophy and less neurological adaptations, among other factors.

It's worth noting that nonfunctional isn't an accurate way to describe this type of muscle building. Sarcoplasmic hypertrophy brings about increases in your ability to store energy and glycogen within the muscle, which of course has a function to play in things like fuel availability. Sarcoplasmic hypertrophy usually occurs more as a result of higher-repetition training methods.

Functional hypertrophy is also known as myofibrillar hypertrophy. The last time you heard about actin and myosin might have been in a high school biology class. These two myofibrillar proteins make up about 20 percent of your muscles. Myosin is the most abundant of these, and an increase in their size and number creates a larger muscle and greater force-producing capabilities (Taber et al. 2019).

If you want your abs to perform and be as strong as they look, you need to train them using progressively heavier weights and a variety of repetition ranges. Hundreds of crunches and hours of plank holds just won't cut it, nor will they cut up your abs!

THREE FACTORS RESPONSIBLE FOR ABDOMINAL GROWTH

It's been suggested that three primary factors are responsible for initiating the muscle growth response (Schoenfeld 2010). Knowing these can help you understand how an exercise works and its usefulness within your training plan.

Mechanical Tension

Mechanical tension is arguably the main factor affecting muscle growth. This is the tension exerted on your muscles to produce, resist, or control force. Mechanical tension is maximized when you're lifting high amounts of resistance with maximal effort. This leads to a high level of muscle fiber recruitment and activation of high-threshold fast motor units. Because the weight is heavy and therefore your speed of movement is slow, these motor units have to exert high force and thus create high levels of mechanical tension.

Mechanical tension is particularly prevalent in methods in which you use a heavy weight, you overload a muscle eccentrically, you hold an isometric position, or you stretch your muscles fully while under tension. Hearing this, you might already be considering which types of exercise are best suited to building your abdominals and other muscles. You might also be visualizing how these exercises feel.

Metabolic Stress

Metabolic stress is another mechanism of great importance, although less so than mechanical tension. Metabolic stress usually comes about as a result of exercise that relies on anaerobic glycolysis for energy production and workouts that are associated with a burning sensation. These workouts produce high levels of lactate and a change in blood pH, which results in this burning sensation. These metabolic byproducts and cellular swelling trigger a surge in anabolic hormones, including human growth hormone and insulin-like growth factors.

Moderate- to lighter-resistance exercises that have more time under tension (TUT), slow repetition training, and any training that gives you an intense muscle pump increases metabolic stress. Research shows that higher-repetition sets trigger more of these metabolic byproducts and therefore metabolic stress as the growth trigger. For example, performing 12 repetitions of three seconds each results in a larger metabolic response than 6 repetitions of six seconds each (Lacerda 2016).

Muscle Damage

Another mechanism for muscle growth is the occurrence of muscle damage. This is often described as a muscle that is damaged repairing itself to become bigger and stronger than before. Although not far from the truth, its importance has been wildly exaggerated.

Muscle fibers generate force through the action of actin and myosin cross-bridge cycling. Actin and myosin are proteins within your muscles that create cross bridges and allow muscle contraction to take place. During resistance training, damage to these and other protein structures occurs. This is especially true during the eccentric phase of contraction. The response to this damage, or microtrauma, can be compared to a muscle strain or even the inflammatory response to an infection. This response is believed to release various growth factors, allowing these proteins and muscles to repair themselves to a bigger and stronger state.

More tissue breakdown is not necessarily better, though. If there's too much tissue breakdown and not enough building of new proteins, muscle volume will not increase. This is what's referred to as a catabolic state in which muscle protein degradation exceeds muscle protein synthesis.

It's important to note that postexercise soreness, or delayed onset muscle soreness (DOMS), is not related to tissue breakdown, but it does accompany exercises and training protocols that cause muscle damage. Although many people chase muscle soreness, it is neither a sign of an effective workout nor essential for muscle development.

Remember that every ab workout should have a specific purpose and goal. The idea behind any workout is to stimulate and not annihilate a muscle. That means that doing more—more exercises, more time spent in the gym, more frequent workouts—is not necessarily better.

Table 1.1 summarizes the key muscle-building mechanisms and types of exercise they are associated with. A mixed training approach that targets all mechanisms to varying degrees will produce the best results.

Table 1.1 Key Muscle-Building Mechanisms and Common Types of Training

Training method	Mechanical tension	Metabolic stress	Muscle damage
Concentric	Lower	Higher	Lower
Eccentric	Higher	Lower	Higher
Isometric	Higher	Higher for longer durations	Higher
High intensity (fewer than 8 reps)	Higher	Lower	Higher
Moderate intensity (8-15 reps)	Moderate	Moderate	Moderate
Low intensity (more than 15 reps)	Lower	Higher	Lower
Intensity techniques (e.g., drop sets, cluster sets)	Higher	Higher	Higher

SHOULD YOUR ABS BE TRAINED DIFFERENTLY?

Common belief is that your abdominal muscles differ from other muscle groups and for that reason should be trained differently. It is often thought that abs require a higher number of repetitions and higher frequency of training than other muscle groups. These beliefs typically stem from several observations. The first is that many people only feel their abs working when using a high number of repetitions. The second is that many people simply don't train their abs in the most efficient way possible. And third, many people believe that the abdominal muscles are endurance-based muscles and should be trained like them.

When you perform a high number of repetitions per set of exercise, you're more likely to feel a burn in the muscle. Many people have a poor connection with their abdominals and, because of inefficient exercise selection and technique, this causes them to chase the burn over anything else. If this is true for you, you won't be blamed for thinking you need a higher number of repetitions to work them harder and get the best results. Instead, the solution is to find better exercises and perfect your execution.

With better exercises and improved body awareness, you'll feel more targeted muscle tension across all repetition ranges. By doing this, you'll achieve far superior results than if you just chase the burn.

Your abs don't require a higher frequency of training than other body parts do. If you aren't working your abs efficiently, then you won't feel much fatigue or soreness, and you won't need much recovery time. The result is feeling as though you could and should train your abs nearly every day. Despite frequent training, this strategy will result in a lack of progress. Instead, the solution comes back to selecting better exercises and perfecting technique and abdominal awareness. When you do this, your training frequency will be less.

Your abdominals are built for a combination of strength, power, and some endurance. They are not solely an endurance muscle. In fact, your abdominals show a mix of type I (slow twitch) and type II (fast twitch) muscle fibers. Across the rectus abdominis and internal and external obliques, proportions of type I fibers range from 55 to 58 percent (Häggmark and Thorstensson 1979). There is some individual variation, but generally, the proportions are relatively even. Compare this to a muscle that *is* built for endurance, the soleus muscle in the calf. This muscle is made up of 60 to 100 percent slow-twitch muscle fibers (Gollnick et al. 1974).

Your abdominals are built for a variety of purposes. Your training should therefore reflect this by including a variety of exercises, methods, training speeds, and repetition ranges.

VOLUME, INTENSITY, AND FREQUENCY OF AB TRAINING

Frequency, volume, and intensity form the foundation of any training program. Whether you're working hard to chisel your abs or grow bigger arms, these three variables matter. They're interrelated, so talking about them together will give you a better understanding so you can apply them to your own training.

Volume

Volume is the total amount of work performed in an individual workout or entire week. When you say that you completed six sets of abs in your workout, you're referring to the total volume of ab work. Studies have shown a linear relationship between muscle growth and increasing the number of reps per muscle group up to about 10 sets per week (Schoenfeld, Ogborn, and Krieger 2016). In other words, doing 10 sets is better than 6 sets, which is better than 3 sets. However, beyond this, results begin to level off. To date, there's no research to say without a doubt that results peak at a certain point.

Individual differences in optimal volume also exist because of genetic and lifestyle factors. While one person might achieve the best results at 22 sets per muscle per week, another may require just 8. In a recent study, participants were split into two groups. In the first group, volume was prescribed to subjects based on the average used in 20 other studies. In this nonindividualized approach, the members of this group each performed the same total volume. In the second group, members were prescribed a volume based on the number of weekly sets they typically completed in their own training. The second training group took a more individualized approach to volume prescription. The results showed that individualized volume led to larger gains than the more generic volume prescribed to the first group (Scarpelli et al. 2020).

A good general recommendation for volume is 10 to 20 sets per muscle group per week (Schoenfeld and Grgic 2017). You should also be willing to experiment. The best way to do this is to keep a detailed training log and assess how your workouts progress over time. You should also monitor things such as your energy levels, sleep, and motivation. Adjust your volume accordingly.

Intensity

Intensity refers to the amount of weight lifted. It's a term often misused to describe how hard someone is working. Technically speaking, it refers to the weight you're lifting and is usually expressed as a percentage of your one repetition maximum (e.g., 75% 1RM). Selecting a weight based on a percentage of your maximum lifting performance can predict the amount of repetitions you can lift with less weight and with great accuracy. Intensity is also at times expressed as a repetition maximum in numbers (e.g., 12 RM). For example, when doing four sets of 10 repetitions at 12RM, the *intensity* is 12RM—the maximum weight you could lift for 12 repetitions.

This is a common error in ab training. The most experienced lifters will program percentages and RMs for the exercises they consider important, yet rarely program their ab exercises. When you consider that your abdominals follow the same laws of human biology as every other muscle in your body, this doesn't make sense. Progressive overload is key, so even spending a little time on correctly programming the intensity of these exercises will take your ab training to the next level.

Intensity directly relates to the number of repetitions you aim to complete in a set. Because training to failure isn't essential, you should select an intensity that allows you to complete each set with one or two repetitions in reserve. This intensity can vary based on several factors, but it is a good general rule to stick with in ab training in particular.

There's an inverse relationship between the amount of resistance you use and the number of repetitions per set. The higher the weight you use (or lower RM), the more sets you will perform. That's because a heavier weight requires fewer repetitions, which require more sets to achieve the same muscle-building stimulus. For example 2 × 20 and 4 × 10 will both create a muscle-building effect, but more repetitions require fewer sets per exercise.

The total number of repetitions you do for each set will be based on those that maximize the development of lean muscle tissue. Hypertrophy studies have shown that muscle can be built using a large variety of repetition ranges (Schoenfeld and Grgic 2017). Based on the available research and how you might best target your abdominals, *most* of your time should be spent in the 8 to 15 repetition range, *some* of your time should also be spent in the 16 to 30 repetition range, and *little* should be spent in the 5 to 7 repetition range (see table 1.2).

Table 1.2 Volume and Intensity Recommendations for Hypertrophy-Based Abdominal Training

Total working sets per week	70% of time spent	20% of time spent	10% of time spent
10-20	8-15 reps, 3-4 sets, 1-2 min rest between sets	16-30 reps, 2-3 sets, 1 min rest between sets	5-7 reps, 4-5 sets, 2-3 min rest between sets

These recommendations might be far from your typical ab workouts. However, your abs follow the same biological principles as every other muscle group does. Of course, performing heavier sets of ab exercises than you're used to might take some time. But don't worry, later chapters will show you exactly how to do this in both a safe and effective manner.

Frequency

Frequency refers to the number of workouts you complete in a week. We won't spend much time on this because the research is pretty clear on the subject: If weekly volume is the same, the total number of workouts you do each week doesn't matter much (Grgic 2018).

To elaborate, the number of workouts you do each week doesn't matter if your total volume is the same and spread between them. We spoke of volume previously and recommended that you do 10 to 20 sets per week for your abs alone. This means that it wouldn't matter if you spread your 10 to 20 sets over six workouts or two of them, for example. Over the six workouts, you might do just one exercise with 3 sets in each (18 sets per week) or two workouts, each with 3 sets of three different exercises (also 18 sets per week). The results would be the same from either approach.

Choose the frequency of workouts that best fits with the rest of your training and according to your own preference. One thing is clear, though: Training frequency per muscle group should occur more than just once per week. Two workouts of 10 sets each will produce better results than one workout of 20 sets. Beyond that, choose whichever ab training frequency suits you best.

EXERCISE SELECTION

Exercise selection is important in any training plan and even more so when training muscles that you might otherwise struggle connecting with. While you might find it easy to squeeze your biceps as hard as you can during a biceps curl, it might not be so easy to feel your abs work during an exercise. There are a variety of reasons for this, and tricks to help you make the connection are discussed later in the book. This is why selecting the best exercises is particularly important for attaining your physique-related goals.

Exercises are tools that provide a stimulus. Selecting the right tools will maximize that stimulus so your abs will grow and become more chiseled. This is also why picking just a few of the right tools, rather than a million and one different ab exercises, will give you far better results. Doing a lot of average exercises with mediocre execution will just lead to average results. Attaining ultimate abs will require more than just being average.

We all have different body types, limb lengths, ranges of motion, and disadvantageous leverages making some exercises more challenging than others. Picking a few exercises that feel good to you is always a good place to start. Focus on exercises in which you can keep the quality high before adding quantity (reps or weight). If you want to build abs, then you need to create an internal focus in every exercise. If you're focused on something outside of your body (the weight you're moving, just completing the reps), then you're missing the point. Make even the lightest sets of that exercise look hard. And, if you don't feel an exercise working where it should be or it's causing pain, then scrap it.

CONSISTENCY OF EXERCISES

Most of what you may have read before will confirm that consistency is important. But what exactly does that mean, and is it really all that important? To some people, the word consistency refers to the act of consistently showing up and staying on top of scheduled workouts. To others, it refers to the consistency of a training plan and repeating the same exercises for a certain number of weeks. While the former is important and deals more with the psychological aspect of training, the latter isn't as cut and dried as some would believe.

Picking the right exercises is key, as you already know. Finding a handful of exercises and progressively overloading these over weeks will also bring about the best results. This involves adding just a few extra repetitions or 1 to 2 percent more weight each week to these exercises. This strategy of progressively overloading your body is guaranteed to work. That being said, you don't want to repeat the exact same exercises for months on end. Not only will progress stall, but it's also a recipe for staleness and training boredom. As a general rule, you shouldn't use the same ab exercises for more than three or four weeks or repeat them over the course of more than six to eight workouts. This will help you overcome a plateau and allow for continued progress.

A recent study found that frequently rotating exercises resulted in greater motivation to work out, compared to repeating the same exercises more consistently. Although the more-consistent study group experienced a learning effect, and bench press strength was slightly better, muscular adaptations were the same. Despite a more randomized rotation of exercises, there were no significant differences between muscle thickness or body composition (Baz-Valle et al. 2019). The results of this study are limited, but they give us a better understanding of the importance of variety in training. While repeating exercises and progressing them over a certain number of weeks are important, there should be rotation within your workouts for the purpose of maintaining motivation. The most practical way to achieve this is to designate priority ab exercises that remain constant until their progress stalls (after three or four weeks), while exercises of less importance can be rotated weekly or even by session (see table 1.3).

Table 1.3 Sample Rotation of Ab Exercises Over a Four-Week Phase of Training

Week 1	Week 2	Week 3	Week 4
Ab wheel rollout	Ab wheel rollout	Ab wheel rollout	Continue to progress or change exercise
Weighted leg raise	Weighted leg raise	Weighted leg raise	Continue to progress or change exercise
Cable crunch	Weighted crunch on ab mat	Sicilian crunch	Vary or return to a previous selection
Kettlebell Russian twist	Cable chop	Resistance band Russian twist	Vary or return to a previous selection

ADHERENCE AND SUSTAINABILITY

Although this book offers many exciting training possibilities that you might be eager to try, if you aren't able to stick to your training plan, then your plan won't work. Although they may seem obvious, three principles underpin the success of any program and deserve discussion.

1. *Realistic:* Your training plan needs to be realistic in terms of your expectations and your time frame. We all want fast results, but this has led many people on a journey of burnout, injury, and lack of long-term progress. In chapter 5, you'll learn about tools for understanding where your body is right now and how to track progress. Understanding where you are can help you create an accurate time frame for real and sustainable progress.

Bodybuilders and physique athletes often have a specific competition date in mind. If they have competed before, they should know how many weeks out they need to start training and dieting. Even if you just want to look great without your shirt on for summer, planning well in advance will give you the best chance of attaining your goals within a manageable time frame. Doing this properly also prevents excessive rebounding of body fat afterward and makes the maintenance of your chiseled abs a whole lot easier. Sustainable summer abs are often made in the winter.

2. *Enjoyable:* For some people, working out feels like an enjoyable hobby. Sure, there are days when it's a struggle, but overall motivation to train is extremely high. For others, it can seem like a daily burden. No matter what workouts are planned or how much spare time they have, they're always thinking of somewhere else they'd rather be. For either personality type, it's important that the workouts and schedule are enjoyable. While some people enjoy trying new exercises or frequently rotating training plans, others find all the enjoyment they need in mastering just a few exercises for a certain number of weeks. Again, personality type matters, and the most important thing should be to experiment and find the approach that works best for you.

Trying to fit to a certain mold will sooner or later cause you to break out, crash, and burn. As a good starting point, try to remain consistent with a handful of key exercises that you enjoy and can feel working. Master those and strive for personal bests. At the same time, exercises of lesser importance can be changed more frequently. There are many other strategies, but this approach can keep the training enjoyable and motivation high.

3. *Flexible:* Your schedule should be flexible and realistic according to the other priorities you already have in your life. It's great getting fired up right now and wanting to crush every exercise you see in this book, but you need a structured way to do it. Work backward and determine how much time you have available to commit. You might think that an optimal training approach would be five or six workouts each week, but what if most weeks you can only do three? Setting expectations too high for your schedule can lead to disappointment when you fail to stick to your plan. The same can be said for thinking you need to spend hours in the gym when realistically you only have a one-hour lunch break to get everything done in. Be realistic not just with your overall goals but your schedule too.

To achieve results on any training plan, you need to be at least 80 percent consistent and compliant. This includes both your training and your diet plan if you're following one. Compliance means that over the course of a month, you miss no more than 20 percent of your scheduled workouts or deviate from the plan no more than 20 percent of the time. If you've deemed 5 workouts each week to be realistic, then you'll do about 20 workouts in a month. If you missed 3 or 4 of these, it wouldn't be a big deal, but more than this would start affecting your progress. Rather than missing more than 20 percent of your training plan, you would be better off designing a plan that calls for fewer workouts. The volume within these fewer workouts would be better suited, and your results would be better. You'd also stress less about missing workouts. When a program is more sustainable it becomes less "I have no life" and more "it's just part of my life."

CONSIDER THE FIVE Ss OF AB-TRAINING OPTIMIZATION

With so much focus on training and diet optimization, it's easy to forget about some of the key lifestyle factors in modern life. These play a large part in optimizing both the performance and recovery from your training and provide the foundation for a healthy and more lifestyle-focused approach. To keep it simple, here are recommendations to ensure you have these five Ss covered.

- **S**leep: Sleep more. Get eight hours whenever possible. Although you might feel fine with less, studies show that very few people can truly optimize with less than six hours.
- **S**tress management: Stress less and relax more. Find strategies that help you switch off. Meditation, relaxing music, and long walks are just a few options. Chewing gum can also take you into a parasympathetic state. This is when your autonomic nervous system puts you in "rest and digest" mode, thereby helping you relax more.
- **S**unlight: Improve hormonal balance and recharge your body. Aim to get outside for 10 to 30 minutes every day. You might need more or less time depending on your region and amount of direct sunlight exposure.
- **S**elf-care: Take care of your body. Don't ignore aches and pains. Get regular massages or use a foam roller frequently.
- **S**upplementation: Use dietary supplements where gaps in your diet need to be filled. Some can aid in sleep, reduce stress, compensate for lack of sunlight, and assist in performance and recovery. Be sure to research them thoroughly.

SUMMARY

We've briefly touched on some of the principles underpinning exercise selection and program design. If you want more information on these principles, a wide variety of textbooks are devoted entirely to them. Having a basic understanding of ab-building principles will help you understand the concepts in the chapters to follow. Next, let's take an even closer look at your abdominals and the important role your spine plays in ab training.

Abdominal and Spinal Anatomy

Before we can talk about how to develop your abs, we have to define what your abs are. We've already mentioned terms such as *six-pack*, *core*, and *muscle activation*, but there's no point in going forward if we can't identify the muscles being targeted.

ABDOMINAL ANATOMY

The core muscles are those that produce and control movement of your lumbar, pelvic, and hip region. These are the muscles of the abdominal wall, back, hip flexors, and glutes. It's an extremely broad term, and you'd likely be surprised by the length of the list of muscles it entails. Don't worry; we won't go into all of them, just the ones you need to know. If you would like to take your anatomy knowledge beyond what is covered in this book there are many educational resources available by searching online.

Of your core, it's your abdominals that we're concerned with. Because your core comprises both deep and superficial muscles, we could also say that it's the superficial abdominals that are of primary focus. That doesn't mean you're superficial, although you're training for six-pack abs here, so you wouldn't be blamed for being just a little; but it's these superficial muscles that are most visible to you in the mirror. Your deep core muscles, on the other hand, are less visible and more responsible for things like spinal stability and maintaining internal abdominal pressure.

The term *abdominals* is generally used to describe four specific muscles that form part of your core musculature: rectus abdominis, transverse abdominis, internal obliques, and external obliques. Let's take a deeper dive into these.

Origins and Insertions

The origins and insertions of muscles are where muscles are attached to your skeleton by connective tissues. To work a muscle effectively, it's important to consider its origins and insertions. Muscles are worked most efficiently when an exercise aligns you in a way that will maximally shorten and lengthen that muscle through its greatest range of motion and with maximal tension.

The rectus abdominis is the superficial six-pack muscle, and it extends the length of the abdomen. It originates from the pubis to insert onto three ribs and sternum. The line down the middle of your six-pack is the linea alba (translated from Latin as *white line*). This is a fibrous structure that separates the rectus abdominis down the middle to create left and right muscle bellies. The linea alba also functions as the attachment site for your other abdominal muscles.

Because we know the placement of the rectus abdominis, we know that to work it fully, we should consider exercises that align and "close the space" between the lower ribs and pubis. Another way to work it is to resist moving the ribs and pelvis farther apart by contracting the rectus abdominis. A handful of exercises might come to mind in both categories—for example, crunches, reverse crunches, and leg raises.

The transverse abdominis (TVA) is a deep muscle that covers a large area of the abdomen and lies beneath the other abdominals. The TVA originates laterally from the lower six ribs, the tensor fasciae latae, and the iliac crest. The iliac crest is the area where arching bones sit on either side of your pelvis. The TVA inserts into the linea alba and a conjoined tendon to your pubis.

Because the TVA is a deep muscle that you can't see, you might think it's not worth training when your goal is appearance, but you'd be wrong. You may not have heard of the Adonis belt (also known as Apollo's belt), but you've probably seen and want one. Way down south, just above your pubic area, are two V-shaped muscular grooves that look like they come up into your obliques. Many consider it one of the most physically attractive features on a man. These lines, technically termed *iliac furrows*, are largely determined by the thickness of your TVA and internal obliques. Therefore, for aesthetic abs, your less visible TVA is important, too.

The external obliques form part of the lateral abdominal wall alongside the internal obliques and TVA. The external obliques are a surface muscle located on either side of your rectus abdominis. They originate from the outer surfaces of the lower eight ribs and insert onto the linea alba and anterior (front) half of the iliac crest.

The external obliques are important visually because they taper down the side of your waist and complement your six-pack abs. By understanding the origins and insertions of the external obliques, we know that spinal lateral flexion (bend to the side) and rotation work best to develop them. The spine is covered in more detail later in the chapter.

The internal obliques are located beneath the external obliques. They originate from the anterior two-thirds of the iliac crest and the lateral half of the inguinal ligament. They insert onto the lower costal connective tissue (cartilage of the eighth to twelfth ribs), the linea alba, and pubic crest (Teyhen et al. 2007). As previously mentioned, the internal obliques form part of the Adonis belt. They might be located under other more visible muscles, but they can have a large visual impact when they're properly developed.

These muscles together form the abdominals. Going forward, the terms *abs*, *abdominals*, and even *six-pack*, refer to these four muscles (see figure 2.1).

Muscle Function

Muscles can only pull from origin to insertion. When we know their attachment sites, we can more clearly understand the function of the abdominals and select better exercises and implement more effective training programs.

Because of its large attachment sites at the pelvis and rib cage, the rectus abdominis acts as the primary flexor of the spine. To work the muscle that gives that six-pack appearance, we *must* pull the pelvis to the rib cage (or vice versa) and flex the spine.

Because of their attachment from the front of the lateral pelvis to the sides of the lower ribs, the external obliques are highly active during spinal rotation and lateral flexion (McGill 1991). To work the obliques in the most efficient way possible, we must perform exercises that involve chopping, rotating, and sideways bending.

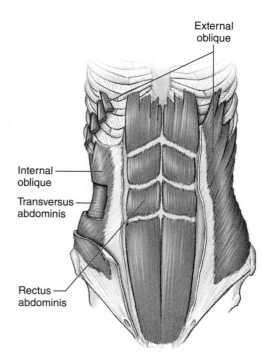

Figure 2.1 Prime abdominal muscles.

Often the muscles of the core are compared to that of a high-pressure cola can. There are a top (diaphragm), bottom (pelvic floor), and sides. This high-pressure and supportive structure functions to stabilize the spine. Because of the origins and insertions of the TVA, we could say that it makes up a large part of the sides of the cola can and holds everything in place. Along with the internal and external obliques, the TVA acts as a key spinal stabilizer. These muscles are reported to contract against the intra-abdominal pressure of the abdominal cavity, thereby increasing stiffness of the lumbar spine against external loads (Teyhen et al. 2007).

The rectus abdominis plays a role in increasing spinal stability, too. Working alongside the erector spinae located at the back, co-contraction with the rectus abdominis increases joint stiffness and spinal stability. Indeed, this "looks only" muscle has an important function to play, too.

The muscles of your core are vast in number. They are key for the efficient functioning of your body. But often when referring to core training, you might actually be referring to your abdominals. These form part of your core and have an important role to play alongside being the muscles you see in the mirror. Core function and training and abs function and training should not be confused. Chapter 3 is devoted to clearing up this confusion and ensuring you're on the right track.

Muscle Function Versus Functional Ab Training

Muscle function and function in the context of training are two different things. They should not be confused, and while one describes the function of a muscle accurately, the other is a term often misunderstood or applied incorrectly to training.

The popularity of so-called functional training has largely driven the core-training craze. At some point, both *functional training* and *core training* became terms used to describe training for six-pack abs. Now here we are today crediting nearly every exercise with working the core. Squats and deadlifts work the core, and it's been proposed that doing these while standing on an unstable surface works the core even more. By this reasoning, maybe we should all be doing wacky circus exercises to develop our abs! Before you head off to find a tightrope, let's rewind and explore ab training in more detail.

Functional training can look like many things to many people. For some, any training performed while balancing on a stability ball can be perceived as functional training. Sure, you're training, but what capacity are you really training? Is this aligned with your visual goals? For others, functional training is any training that mimics an athletic movement almost exactly, usually with the inclusion of a small amount of extra load or velocity; an overweighted baseball bat comes to mind. We won't go down *that* rabbit hole though.

Functional training is simply any training method that will develop a person's ability to function at a given task or sporting activity. If a training plan enhances an elderly person's ability to get out of bed in the morning, then they have trained functionally. If an exercise helps you run faster, jump higher, or throw a ball farther, that exercise is functional for that task.

Some exercises are more functional than others because they transfer to a larger number of movements. Other exercises have little carryover. If an exercise targets a specific muscle, then that exercise enhances that muscle's function. It will help it better *do* what it was designed to. Now that you understand what functional exercise is, let's take another step forward.

Core training might be considered more functional to some people because it requires many muscles to work together. This will be discussed in more detail in the next chapter. For now, consider one of the most popular so-called functional core exercises.

A plank is typically performed with your elbows on the floor. Visualizing this position, is the plank functional according to the definition of functional training? Apart from a plank being functional in its ability to get better at performing a plank, it's likely you can't think of many scenarios in which this position transfers to other tasks. That's not to pick on planks and say that they're useless but merely to provoke thought.

Any exercise can be deemed functional if it trains a muscle's ability to produce force in a way that transfers to something. That exercise might also be deemed more functional if it trains those muscles in an integrated way because muscles don't typically work in isolation in real life. Functional training should therefore be considered as a continuum rather than stating simply that something either *is* or *isn't* functional. The continuum should be based on what the training is trying to be functional *for* (see figure 2.2). Whether something is functional or not also has nothing to do with how effective that exercise is for developing six-pack abs.

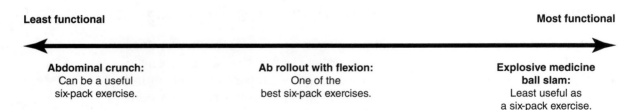

Figure 2.2   Theoretical progression and continuum of functional ab training for an athlete who uses an overhead-throwing motion.

The rectus abdominis is involved in flexion of the spine. It is also responsible for some spinal stability. Those are its functions. So, training your rectus abdominis could be said to be functional for any movement in which spinal flexion is important. How about sitting up and getting out of bed in the morning? What about throwing a ball from an overhead position—for example, a throw-in in soccer? Both of these tasks and many more require strength from your rectus abdominis. And while there are integrated exercises that train them, in order to build a solid strength foundation, an element of isolation is needed. In other words, selecting exercises that activate the rectus abdominis the most will not only help you develop six-pack abs but also improve your function and athleticism. This is the same for your abdominals (see table 2.1).

Table 2.1 Know Your Abdominals

Muscle	Location	Movement	Related function	Example exercise types
Rectus abdominis	Superficial	Flexion of the spine Some trunk stability	Moving from lying to sitting Throwing a ball Looking good	Crunch Leg raise Ab rollout
External obliques	Superficial	Rotation Lateral flexion Some trunk stability	Twisting Golf swing Looking good	Cable chop Russian twist Side bend
Transverse abdominis	Deep	Trunk stability	Posture Intra-abdominal pressure Support of internal organs	Most to some degree
Internal obliques	Deep	Trunk stability Some lateral flexion	Posture Intra-abdominal pressure Support of internal organs	Most to some degree

AB ACTIVATION
DURING DIFFERENT TYPES OF EXERCISE

Understanding muscle activation and what affects it is important when training to build your body. Knowing what types of exercise produce the greatest levels of activation allows you to identify the exercises best suited to your goals.

Muscle Testing and Electromyography

Among exercise scientists, it's widely accepted that electromyography (EMG) testing is a useful way to determine levels of muscle activation. The levels of muscle activation achieved during an exercise can determine the effectiveness of that exercise for targeting specific muscles. In our case, we're most concerned with exercises that produce the highest levels of activation in the abdominal muscles.

From chapter 1, we know that isometric contractions are when muscles produce tension without changing their length or resulting in a change in joint angle. Maximal voluntary contraction (MVC) is a measurement of how hard a muscle can contract isometrically. When exercise scientists test MVC, they do so by putting you in an advantageous position and ask you to contract your abs as hard as you can. Using electromyography, an exercise scientist can test an exercise and provide a percentage of activation comparable to MVC; the activation achieved in the exercise is compared to when you simply contract. This is why we often see numbers surpassing 100 percent MVC, but it's also why it's difficult to compare one study directly to another because testing protocols aren't standardized.

Electromyography can be used to test both *peak* and *mean* muscle activation. Exercise scientists often use mean MVC for their data, which shows the average muscle activation through an entire repetition. Unfortunately, this doesn't always give the full story of the exercise. While some exercises produce high levels of activation, they may do so for a very short period of time. Other exercises might produce lower levels of peak activation but for a longer amount of time.

Different exercises have different muscle activation profiles. One exercise might be great at achieving high levels of peak activation in one position (e.g., the top of an abdominal crunch), while another might be very good at achieving high levels of peak activation in another position (e.g., the bottom of an ab rollout). So considering both mean and peak muscle activation is important. Peak activation can be used to determine the most effective portion of an exercise, while exercises that show high levels of mean activation might be better for creating a pump-type effect within the muscle. We'll take this into account throughout the book.

Compound Exercises

Performing only heavy compound exercises like squats and deadlifts is far from an optimal strategy for attaining six-pack abs. A handful of studies have assessed abdominal activation during these compound exercises. The rectus abdominis and external obliques display moderate levels of muscle activation, at best, during heavy back squats and deadlifts. Both the squat and deadlift also produce similar levels of TVA muscle activation (Hamlyn, Behm, and Young 2007; Willardson, Fontana, and Bressel 2009).

Strongman Exercises

During strongman-type exercises, rectus abdominis muscle activity is also moderate, although higher levels of activation can be achieved in the tire flip and Atlas stone lift (about 69 to 87 percent of maximal voluntary contraction). To put that into perspective, it's not uncommon for some ab exercises to achieve well beyond 100 percent rectus abdominis activation using comparative testing methods. External oblique activation during strongman exercises is higher. These show up to 103 percent during Atlas stone lifts and 106 percent during tire flips (McGill, McDermott, and Fenwick 2009).

Unstable Exercises

Exercises performed on a stability ball and other unstable surfaces can show moderate to high levels of abdominal muscle activation, which is more than when using body weight alone. In a study comparing traditional ab exercises on the floor to those performed on a stability ball, the curl-up (crunch) performed on a stability ball achieved higher levels of rectus abdominis activation than when it was performed on the floor (Duncan 2009). In a similar study also with a crunch variation, using a stability ball showed no added benefit to rectus abdominis activation, although higher activation was seen in the external obliques when a stability ball was used (Imai et al. 2010).

A study comparing a basic body-weight plank to using a stability ball and suspension trainer showed that the suspension trainer achieved the highest levels of rectus abdominis activation. Although it significantly outperformed other plank variations, only moderate levels of activation were achieved (Atkins et al. 2015). It's important to note that these studies used body weight alone, and while overall it appears as though there's no downside to using unstable surfaces to maximally activate your abdominals, it's likely that using unstable surfaces reduce your ability to perform weighted ab exercises. In other words, using unstable surfaces may be better than the floor alone during exercises such as crunches, but it may be better to stick to the floor and progress to doing exercises faster and with resistance. This is purely speculative, though.

Isometric and Dynamic Exercises

When comparing isometric to dynamic exercises, we see a clear difference in abdominal muscle activation. Rectus abdominis and oblique muscle activation is higher during dynamic exercises such as rollouts and pike-to-plank variations than during a standard plank exercise. When comparing exercises, rollouts, pikes, and even sit-up and crunch variations almost always come out on top (Aspe and Swinton 2014; Stenger 2013).

Muscle activation will continue to be a theme in part II. It's one way to determine how effectively an exercise targets a certain portion of your abdominals. I'll also share tips for enhancing muscle activation in exercises you might already be doing—for example, how to activate your abs up to 26 percent more during ab rollouts. In chapter 3 we'll take an in-depth look at the exercises themselves.

SPINAL ANATOMY

When talking about ab training and exercises we must discuss the spine (see figure 2.3). We've already used terminology related to the spine and will continue to do so throughout this book. The following section briefly explores spinal anatomy and defines concepts and terminology used later in the book.

Spinal flexion exercises have become a contentious subject in the fitness and scientific community. As we explore the functional anatomy of the spine, you will be better positioned to decide for yourself whether exercises such as crunches and those that involve flexing your spine are "bad" for you.

Your spine is the central support system for your entire body. It assists in some way with nearly every movement you make, provides a structure that contributes to protection of your internal organs, and supports your spinal cord. It needs to be strong enough to hold your body weight when standing and resist being subjected to large forces. It also needs to be flexible enough to allow for movement. It's an impressive piece of craftsmanship and an important one at that.

Your spine consists of 33 vertebrae. These are connected by facet joints that link your skull to your pelvis. Your facet joints allow the vertebrae to glide smoothly

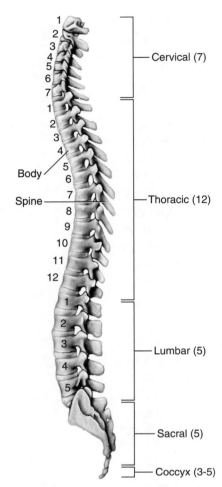

Figure 2.3 Anatomy of the spine showing cervical, thoracic, lumbar, sacral, and coccygeal regions.

against each other and for the spine to flex, extend, and rotate. Each vertebra has three main components:

1. The vertebral body at the back of each of your vertebra supports your body weight.
2. The vertebral arch at the front of the vertebra protects your spinal cord.
3. The spinous and transverse processes around the back and toward the sides of each vertebra serve as sites that the ligaments to attach to.

All but nine vertebrae are moveable, and these are divided into three groups:

1. The cervical, or neck, region (7 vertebrae)
2. The thoracic, or midback, region (12 vertebrae)
3. The lumbar, or lower-back, region (5 vertebrae)

The sacral (5 vertebrae) and coccygeal (3-5 vertebrae, depending on individual anatomy) groups are fused together and do not move.

Cervical Spine

The cervical spine (your neck) is made up of the first seven vertebrae and is shaped like an inward C, called a lordotic curve. Your cervical region is strong enough to hold the entire weight of your head (13-20 lb [6-9 kg]). It is also the most flexible part of your spine and allows head and neck movement to take place. Cervical flexion is dropping your chin to your chest; normal range of motion (ROM) is about 45 degrees. Cervical extension is lifting your chin and looking up; normal ROM is about 45 degrees. In lateral flexion, your ear drops to the side toward your shoulder, and ROM is also about 45 degrees. Looking left and right requires cervical rotation, and about 80 degrees is available in each direction. Unless you are performing abdominal exercises with poor technique, there shouldn't be much movement of your neck. Because of its natural structure, neck training will make it stronger and more stable.

Thoracic Spine

The thoracic spine (your midback) is made up of 12 vertebrae and is shaped like a backward C called a kyphotic curve. It's the largest portion of your spine, and its primary function is to protect your organs in the chest cavity by holding your rib cage in place. Of course, having a rib cage is a good thing, but it's also what limits the thoracic portion of your spine from flexing and extending. As a result, your thoracic spine is largely geared toward rotation. When performing a chopping-type exercise, for example, some movement can take place at the thoracic region of your spine. Because of its naturally limited ROM in certain directions, maintaining and improving thoracic mobility through training is important.

Lumbar Spine

The lumbar spine (your lower back) is a mobile portion of the vertebral column. The inward C shape, or arch in your lower back, is referred to as a lordotic curve. This region has five vertebrae and sits below the thoracic region. Together with the thoracic spine, it allows the most spinal movement to take place. When flexing and bending forward, roughly 90 degrees of ROM are available. Lateral flexion (bending to the side), rotation, and extension of combined lumbar and thoracic regions allow approximately 30 degrees of ROM. Because of its natural structure, the lumbar region requires training to make it more stable. This includes developing dynamic strength through different ranges of motion as well as the ability to resist movement.

Sacrum and Coccyx

The sacrum (hip complex) is made up of five fused vertebrae, meaning it's relatively immoveable. Instead, these sacral vertebrae are important for stabilizing other bones and muscles around your lumbar–pelvic and hip region. The coccygeal vertebrae are at the end of your spine and form your coccyx, often referred to as the tail bone. Because of its structure, training of this area should focus on strength and stability of the muscles around it and mobility of the sacroiliac joint (located between the sacrum and ilium bones of the pelvis) and hip joint.

SPINAL STABILITY AND MOBILITY

Spinal stability refers to how well one can maintain a certain spinal position in the presence of change. For example, when holding a heavy grocery bag in one hand, a stable spine keeps the weight of the bag from pulling you into a side bend, or lateral flexion. Your abdominals, and particularly your obliques, help stabilize your spine in that scenario. Mobility, on the other hand, refers to what a joint can do on its own and without influence. Your spine is designed to be stable and move well in all directions.

The spine has many functions. It also has limitations. A joint-by-joint approach to exercise selection takes into consideration these functions and limitations (see figure 2.4). The model at its simplest asks this question: Are you mobile where you should be mobile and are you strong and stable where you should be? These are important considerations in spine and abdominal training.

THE ANTICRUNCH MOVEMENT

If you've been wandering the fitness forums and other outlets over the past decade, you likely have been taken on a rollercoaster ride of abdominal training recommendations. If we start from the 1980s and go into the 1990s, most ab training was based on flexing and twisting motions. Your favorite movie action heroes weren't balancing on a stability ball. They were doing sit-ups and leg raises. Maybe their abs were being tenderized by boxing gloves, too, but that's about as fancy as it got.

Years later—it's difficult to say exactly when—so-called functional core training started to appear. Possibly it grew out of sit-up and crunch boredom, or maybe something else challenged the industry's beliefs. Any fitness media outlet that

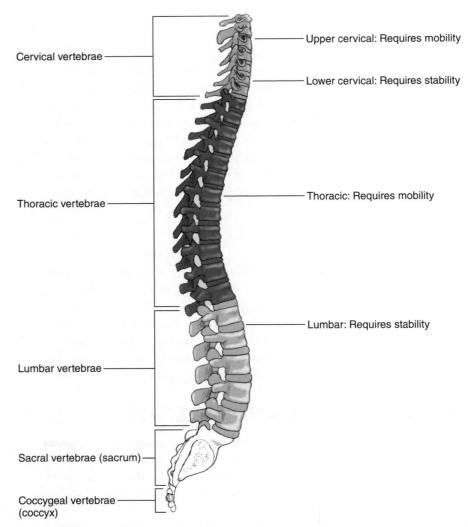

Cervical vertebrae

Upper cervical: Requires mobility

Lower cervical: Requires stability

Thoracic vertebrae

Thoracic: Requires mobility

Lumbar: Requires stability

Lumbar vertebrae

Sacral vertebrae (sacrum)

Coccygeal vertebrae
(coccyx)

Figure 2.4   Regions of the spine showing an alternating series of stability and mobility segments.

didn't have "core" written on the front page or a plank variation inside would probably have gone broke. *Core* was used largely as a marketing term and became synonymous with your abs and having a healthy and functional body. Anything that involved flexing your spine, and especially performing exercises like crunches, was considered bad for you. Full stop; no questions asked.

The belief that crunches and similar flexion-based exercises were "bad" largely stemmed from a small number of back-pain specialists questioning their use (McGill 2010). These concerns were usually predicated on the belief that the spine has only a certain number of bending cycles, and beyond this, damage to the spinal discs will start to take place (McGill 2017). This information spread fast and became a popular belief among strength and conditioning coaches. Because of the incorrect application of functional training, everything meshed to form an anticrunch mentality. Flexion-based exercises in isolation were often considered useless (Schuler and Cosgrove 2010).

Today the tables are turning. Fitness professionals are coming around to the belief that there's a place for both schools of thought. While performing largely isometric exercises and integrated core movements can be most effective for achieving some goals, ab exercises that involve flexing and rotating are important for other goals—different horses for different courses.

For the sole purpose of achieving six-pack abs, training them in isolation and according to their designed function—the rectus abdominis is designed to flex the spine—is the most efficient and effective way. For the purposes of sport and transfer to multijoint exercises and movements, multijoint ab and core exercises should also be used. Remember though, the more time and attention you can commit to exercises that are best suited for abdominal hypertrophy the faster you'll get abs. All other goals should be secondary to that.

IS SPINAL FLEXION "BAD"?

We've already gone into some of the benefits of including isolation and, in particular, the exercises that involve spinal flexion. With the high levels of muscle activation alone, the benefits to your six-pack abs are clear. It's therefore the risk that we need to consider in more depth.

Will crunches and similar exercises help you get six-pack abs, but at the expense of your back health? The short answer is no. But let's look into this a little deeper and use science and sense to answer it.

This is a question that plagues the minds of many fitness professionals, especially those who train high-level athletes. Strength coaches wouldn't want to risk their athletes getting awesome abs at the expense of their careers. That just wouldn't go down well at the head office. For many coaches, the perceived risk outweighs the reward of certain ab exercises (Schuler and Cosgrove 2010).

Proponents of the "spinal flexion is bad" theory recommend limiting the bending of the spine to essential daily activities, such as tying your shoelaces. Exercises like crunches are therefore considered unnecessary and unsafe. Concerns about spinal flexion are usually based on the belief that the spine has a finite number of bending cycles, as we previously mentioned. It's proposed that exceeding these bending cycles causes damage to the spinal discs. Back in 2011, in a thorough review of the research available at the time, a paper examining the potential risks and applicability of spinal flexion exercises concluded that

The claim that dynamic flexion exercises are injurious to the spine in otherwise healthy individuals remains highly speculative and is based largely on the extrapolation of in vitro animal data that is of questionable relevance to in vivo human spinal biomechanics. (Contreras and Schoenfeld 2011)

In other words, a paper written by experienced and highly educated coaches and researchers, that went through a thorough peer-review process and was analyzed by other highly educated researchers and was printed in one of the most respected strength and conditioning journals concluded that there is no evidence that exercises such as crunches cause damage to your spine.

Much of the original research was done on the spines of pigs, and not living ones at that. It is this research that was popularized and spread the word that spinal flexion was bad. First off, you are not a pig. And unlike a pig, you walk upright, which has bearings on how your spine is built and deals with load. Second, you are alive. You are composed of living tissue that adapts according to targeted stress—the same type of stress we spoke about in chapter 1 that helps you build muscle and has many other benefits. This commonly referenced original research left out the question of how our spines adapt over time when subjected to progressive strengthening of the abdominals and using a variety of spine movements.

A range of exercises are required to work your abdominals effectively. These exercises will differ according to your training objectives. Using a large variety of abdominal exercises will also vary spinal loading, while complementary exercises to your abdominal workouts can even work to unload the spine. Changing the way you load your spine is associated with a lower risk of spinal pathology (Videman, Nurminen, and Troup 1990).

SUMMARY

I'll conclude by stating the position of this book on flexion-based exercises: The goal of this book is to help you build an aesthetic and chiseled set of abdominal muscles. To do that, you should use the best exercises, those with the research and real-world results to back them up. I also don't want to recommend exercises that have a high risk factor and affect your long-term progress. To be clear, I am not necessarily recommending that simple abdominal crunches are the best. Instead, what I am suggesting is that exercises like crunches and those that involve dynamic motions of the spine can have profound benefits to your six-pack training when applied correctly. According to the available evidence, dynamic flexions of the spine pose no risk to an otherwise healthy back. This book offers a large variety of the exercises to help you meet your primary objective.

Ab Versus Core Training

In chapter 2, we discussed abdominal anatomy, and we also touched on the core. In this chapter, we discuss the difference between core and ab training in detail from both an anatomical and training standpoint so you will be able to formulate an effective strategy without losing sight of your ultimate goal of six-pack abs. Achieving chiseled abs alongside a strong and functional core is indeed attainable, and I'll share strategies for working toward both. However, the more time and attention you can focus initially on aesthetics, the better results you'll get while also building a foundation for future and more performance-based goals. This book takes you through a journey of learning exercises that will allow you to achieve this. But first, this chapter explains the differences between ab training and core training and how blending them can produce the most impressive results.

THE CORE

Definitions of core training and core anatomy are wide and varied, so it's no wonder we often lose sight of what we're training. If professionals and the scientific community can't agree on exactly what the core is, then how are you supposed to? You can't target what you don't know.

Definition

As we learned in chapter 2, the core includes any muscle and structure that produces and controls movement around the lumbo–pelvic–hip complex, which consists of musculoskeletal structures that stabilize the spine and pelvis. Simply put, your core comprises an awful lot, including muscles and connective tissues (tendons, fascia) that influence your spine and pelvis.

From an aesthetic standpoint, we're mostly concerned with the muscles. The core muscles include your glutes, deep multifidi and intercostal muscles, and even your latissimus dorsi (lats). The deep multifidi are part of the transversospinalis group of muscles that are small muscles located around the spine that help support and produce movement. The intercostals are also a group of small muscles, but run between your ribs and have an important role to play within breathing mechanics. The latissimus dorsi is a large back muscle that essentially connects your upper arm to your lower back and pelvis, but it is often not thought of as part of your core. Although your hamstrings also influence your pelvis, a line must be drawn, and they are not considered part of the core. And yes, your core muscles also include your abdominals (see table 3.1).

Table 3.1   Key Core Muscles (Including Those Identified as Abdominals With Checkmark Symbol)

Core muscle	Abdominal muscle
Erector spinae	
Multifidus	
Quadratus lumborum	
Gluteus maximus	
Gluteus minimus	
Gluteus medius	
Latissimus dorsi	
Muscles of the neck	
Rectus abdominis	✓
Transverse abdominis	✓
External obliques	✓
Internal obliques	✓
Muscles of the pelvic floor	
Hip flexors	

Core Versus Abdominals

Of your entire core musculature, only four of these muscles are said to be part of your abdominals. And of your abdominals, only two of those are visible. In chapter 2, we discussed the benefits of training your deep internal obliques and transverse abdominis (TVA) from a visual perspective and to develop your Adonis belt, but only your rectus abdominis and external obliques are truly visible.

You might be thinking that focusing on core training would be most beneficial because it hits the most muscle mass. And you'd be right, it *can* be. Training your core means working everything that controls your spine and pelvis, teaching it to function as one unit. There are benefits to this both from a functional perspective and for health-based objectives. Working a larger amount of muscle also means you burn more calories and get a greater hormonal response. Both are good things, especially when trying to optimize your overall body chemistry to get lean and build muscle. But your goals are clear, and to get six-pack abs you need to focus on your priorities.

Let's use an example of trying to build sleeve-popping biceps. If you use "big muscle mass" exercises like pull-ups, sure, your biceps will get a workout. But for most, these exercises alone aren't enough to put a significant amount of mass on your arms. Pull-ups can form part of the program, but more biceps-focused exercises are essential for reaching your goal of achieving big biceps.

Training for six-pack abs is the same. Core exercises are to your abs as pull-ups are to your biceps, and ab-focused exercises are the equivalent of the biceps curl. Blending both approaches will produce the best results. Although exercises that are integrated and hit your core as a unit are included in this book, focused ab exercises are also essential for targeting that area. Choose exercises that are core focused based on how effectively they target your abdominals rather than your core overall.

The core exercises spotlighted later in this book have been included or adapted based on how effectively they work your abdominals. An approach that blends exercises higher on the functional continuum with exercises that produce the most muscle activation will produce the most impressive results.

CORE EXERCISES AND TRAINING

Core training primarily focuses on the development of core and spinal stability. Spinal stability refers to how well you can maintain a certain spinal position in the presence of change. We touched on this in chapter 2, and using our definition of the core, this can be further extended to the pelvis. When an external force comes into play, your spine and pelvis need to be able to maintain their position. If they are not, they are more prone to acute or chronic injury or excessive wear and tear. This is vastly important from a health perspective. From a performance perspective it's important too, because if you can resist an external force, you're not only less likely to get injured or crushed by an opponent, you're also in a better position to express force in the opposite direction. The better you can absorb, the more you can give back.

Resisting change can also be described as being able to fight against or oppose change. A term often used to describe core exercises is *antiexercises*: antiextension, antirotation, and so on. *Anti* means to oppose something, which in this case is the position of your spine or pelvis in the presence of change. Chapter 10 will cover antimovements in more detail, but for now consider core exercises as those with the purpose of developing a stable spine and pelvis by *resisting* movement. Examples of this include the following:

• *Resisting lumbar extension and anterior pelvic tilt (APT) during a plank:* A traditional front plank is an example of such an event. Positioning a weight on your lumbar region applies an additional force, and if it's not resisted, it takes you farther into lumbar extension and anterior pelvic tilt—your pelvis tilting forward. It is the job of the muscles that create a pulling force in the opposite direction (lumbar flexion, posterior pelvic tilt) to resist lumbar extension and APT. From our discussion of abdominal anatomy, you know that your rectus abdominis in particular plays a large role here as well as other muscles working in unity.

• *Resisting lateral flexion of the spine and lateral hip movement while carrying heavy groceries:* Every time you carry a bag in one hand or pick up a suitcase this is happening. Swapping that heavy grocery bag for an even heavier dumbbell and performing a one-handed farmer's carry applies an additional force that, if not resisted, would pull you farther into spinal lateral flexion and hip adduction (towards the midline of the body). Moving the weight farther from your center of mass increases the challenge too. Your TVA, internal and external obliques, quadratus lumborum (located on either side of your back abdominal wall), and glutes would work hard to resist these forces. If they didn't, you'd crumble.

• *Resisting spinal rotation when holding a cable during a chopping movement:* These movements might be difficult to visualize now, but you'll see excellent examples in chapters 9 and 10. The cable Pallof press is one of them. The greater the resistance coming from the cable, the greater the challenge of being rotated toward it. When the cable is held closer to your body, it is easier. Pressing the cable farther away makes it more difficult. Your obliques on the opposing side and TVA fire like crazy to resist and work with a host of other muscles around your spine and pelvis. There are plenty of scenarios in which you need to resist spinal rotation in both sporting and daily activities.

The previous examples are simple and don't tell the full story of what's going on. Many movements—both big and small—are being resisted, and a lot of muscles and other structures are being challenged. You now have a picture of what a core-focused training plan works toward.

CORE VERSUS AB EXERCISES AND TRAINING

Core exercises should be seen and programmed according to movements that relate to specific functional tasks. When selecting a core exercise for your program, you should be able to justify it in the following way:

> *"I'm using (exercise name) to train my ability to resist (spinal or pelvic movement), which will help (daily or sporting task)."*

This might look something like the following:

> *"I'm using the dead-bug exercise to train my ability to resist rotation of my spine and pelvis, which will help improve my running economy."*

In this scenario, the dead bug, which can be an effective exercise for a variety of purposes, is considered a useful and functional exercise for runners training their core.

Ab training and exercise selection are muscle focused. Although we might understand the movement that is taking place (e.g., spinal flexion in an abdominal crunch), we might not necessarily choose that exercise for its ability to transfer to a particular daily or sporting task. A strong muscle will contribute to this transfer, but primarily we're concerned with how that muscle looks. When selecting an ab exercise for your program, you should be able to justify it in the following way:

> *"I'm using (exercise name) to maximally target my (abdominal muscle name)."*

This might look something like the following:

> *"I'm using ab wheel rollouts to maximally target my rectus abdominis."*

By now the difference between core and ab training should be clear. Because your goals are centered mostly on aesthetics, taking an ab-focused training approach will produce the best results. Secondary to that, core training should also be included for the other benefits outside of aesthetics. By blending ab and core training, you'll develop an impressive set of abs that not only look good but perform just as well. This approach also adds variety to your routines so that developing ultimate abs is an enjoyable process.

THE BEST AB EXERCISES ACCORDING TO RESEARCH

Not every abdominal and core exercise has a research paper behind it. But to some degree, science has done a good job of directing us in the right direction when it comes to selecting the best exercises to target certain areas of your abdominals. Here's what some of the research has to say.

Sit-Ups

Sit-ups have a role to play in an ultimate ab program. I wouldn't mention them here if they didn't. Bent-knee and extended-knee sit-up exercises have been shown to be effective in activating the rectus abdominis and internal and external obliques (Juker et al. 1998). They also achieve high levels of muscle activation in your hip flexors (particularly the rectus femoris), which can cause problems for some people. There is a relationship between dominant hip flexors and back pain. In this case, modified versions of sit-ups are an effective solution (Sullivan 2015). They also help "switch off" your hip flexors by recruiting other muscles (Larson et al. 2007). These strategies are covered in chapter 7. Therefore, while some abdominal exercises are excellent at targeting your abdominals, you need to consider whether they also activate other muscles you might not want to activate for various reasons.

Crunch Variations

Traditional crunches and their derivatives can be a useful addition to your ab-building toolbox, as long as they're done correctly. Studies consistently show that crunches can achieve respectable levels of muscle activation targeted to your abdominals, particularly your rectus abdominis six-pack muscle. This makes sense because they work directly according to the function of the rectus abdominis in pulling your ribs toward your pelvis. Crunches are also frequently recommended in place of sit-ups. This is because crunches can activate your abdominals just as effectively as sit-ups can, but without the relatively high hip flexor activation (Guimaraes et al. 1991). Crunches can be performed in a variety of ways and using different devices. Crunch variations can include lying on the floor or on a stability ball, using weights, or even kneeling and crunching with a cable. One thing is clear, though: Your abdominals produce greater levels of activation when crunches are performed with added resistance (Moraes 2009). The intricacies of each of these variations are described in chapter 7.

Reverse Crunches and Leg Raises

The lower portion of your rectus abdominis is a notoriously hard place to hit. If you want six- or even eight-pack abs, then this area needs to be developed. The most effective exercises are those that focus on performing what's referred to as a posterior pelvic tilt (PPT), in which the pelvis tilts backward. The function of the rectus abdominis is to pull the ribs to the pelvis, or in the case of reverse crunches, think of them as pulling your pelvis up toward your ribs. This tilt of the pelvis is the PPT we're referring to, and it preferentially recruits the lower portion of your six-pack (Sarti et al. 1996). When considering pelvis position independently, it has been shown that the highest rectus abdominis activation can be achieved in a PPT position (Workman et al. 2008). Reverse crunches performed on a decline and leg raise variations can reap significant benefits when proper progression takes place.

Pikes and Knee Tucks

Pikes and knee tucks can be performed using a stability ball, suspension trainer, or even core sliders. While knee tucks are done with a bend of the knees, pikes are done with a straighter leg and are a progression of the former. Both knee tucks and pikes focus on achieving a PPT while resisting lumbar extension in the bottom positions, and they can achieve high levels of muscle activation in your abdominals (Escamilla et al. 2006; Escamilla, Lewis, and Bell 2010). While pikes show greater activation, this does not necessarily mean they are better than knee tucks. It is especially important for beginners to progress these exercises correctly. Both exercises are considered core exercises because they recruit a large amount of muscle mass beyond the abdominals. Solely as an abdominal exercise, they're highly effective, and for this reason they're a valuable exercise in the development of both an aesthetic and resilient midsection.

Ab Rollouts

In a 2017 study examining four common ab exercises performed on a suspension trainer, rollouts and body saws came out on top (Cugliari and Boccia 2017). Electromyography (EMG) data showed higher levels of rectus abdominis and oblique activation in rollouts than in pikes and knee tucks. In a study examining 12 nontraditional ab exercises, ab rollouts performed best for the lower abdominal region, second best for upper abdominals, and a respectable fourth place for external obliques (Escamilla et al. 2006). The ab wheel rollout consistently performed well, while 11 other ab exercises showed large differences in the area of the abs they activated. For example, the same study found that for the upper rectus abdominis, a reverse crunch inclined to 30 degrees was the best. For the lower rectus abdominis the rollout came out on top, with hanging knee raises and pikes second and third. For the obliques, the pike came out on top. In this particular study, only 12 exercises were tested, but of these, the majority had been shown to perform well in previous studies. Overall, rollouts outperformed a lot of stiff competition. A 2010 study (Escamilla, Lewis, and Bell 2010) compared 8 exercises performed on a stability ball. The study showed that both rollouts and pikes done on a stability ball were most effective for targeting the upper and lower rectus abdominis and external and internal obliques while also minimizing muscle activation in unwanted areas (lumbar paraspinals, rectus femoris). With that in mind, you'll find a variety of pike and rollout variations throughout chapters 7, 8, and 10.

Rotational Crunches and Twisting Sit-Ups

Crunches and sit-ups incorporating twisting motions are commonly believed to be good for targeting your obliques and can preferentially recruit that area of the abdominals. However, it's interesting that exercises like ab rollouts, pikes, and even hanging knee raises activate the external obliques more than twisting crunch variations do (Escamilla et al. 2006). A variation of a twisting crunch, a bicycle crunch, has been shown to produce greater external oblique activation than a side plank (Stenger 2013). While that may be true, in the same study a front plank outperformed a side plank in external oblique activation. So it's really not that impressive after all. In this same study, the top performers for external oblique activation were rollouts, hanging leg raises, and reverse crunches. Considering the levels of overall abdominal activation achieved by other exercises, one has to question whether twisting crunches and sit-ups are worth it. With a few tweaks they *can* be. Some loaded variations deserve a place in this book, but only as assistance exercises to those that offer better results.

Chopping Exercises

One of the functions of your core is to transfer force from your lower to upper body. Look at athletes in action, and it's clear to see when this is happening. Your entire core plays an active role in rotational strength and power in movements like throwing, turning, swinging a golf club, grappling, and punching. If you want to improve at these and develop a core that performs at high levels, the principle of specificity dictates that chopping-type exercises be included in your routine. They're great for teaching your lower and upper body to work together to produce rotation. Chopping-type motions can be considered functional exercises for this purpose. They can also be useful for increasing mobility in the thoracic spine and hips. Although EMG studies using these exercises are limited, it makes sense that they're useful for activation of the internal and external obliques as well as the TVA. To develop abs that both perform and look good, chopping exercises should be in your routine.

Planks and Long-Lever Plank Variations

Plank variations are generally considered to be core focused because they're used to target a large number of muscles. We've already discussed how they stand up as a core and ab exercise. The traditional front plank offers your abdominal development very little. And according to our definition of functional training (see chapter 2), planks don't transfer much to activities other than planks themselves. That being said, we cannot ignore their use as a potential beginner exercise or one that will transfer to an effective position during push-ups. Compared to the traditional front plank, an exercise that *is* worth using is the long-lever posterior-tilt plank. Besides the much longer name, it also wins for its ability to produce greater levels of activation in the rectus abdominis, lower abdominal stabilizers, and external obliques (Schoenfeld et al. 2014). On top of long-lever planks, loaded versions holding a posteriorly tilted pelvis warrant use, too. Using a suspension trainer to perform planks can increase abdominal activation (Byrne et al. 2014), while even the position of your shoulder blades can be manipulated in order to activate your abdominals further (Cortell-Tormo 2017). Isometric exercises like the plank can be useful, but it's important that they be challenging. You have a lot of options for upgrading your regular old front planks to make them work better. Chapter 10 will offer options.

Bird Dogs and Dead Bugs

They might have weird names, but these exercises can be an important part of an ab training program, and injury prevention and functional performance are secondary goals. These exercises train the ability of your spine and pelvis to resist rotation. Overall abdominal activation is relatively low in these at the basic level, but this can vary depending on technique and even the speed at which you perform them (Yun et al. 2017). When doing these exercises, much like a plank, basic body-weight versions should be reserved for complete beginners or those with rehabilitation goals in mind. Creative ways to load dead bugs and bird dogs are required to make them more effective (see chapter 10). As a primary exercise to develop six-pack abs, these are disappointing, but to help prevent injury and increase spinal and pelvic stability, these are some of the best.

Pallof Presses and Other Antirotation Exercises

The Pallof press is an old exercise that's recently become more popular as a means to improve rotational core strength as a part of rehabilitation programs and to improve back health. These exercises can be effective, especially when progressed to use considerable amounts of resistance. Pallof presses aren't generally used for aesthetic purposes, but they could be a good option for developing the Adonis belt mentioned in chapter 2. Similar to Pallof presses, standing one-arm cable presses offer many of the same benefits in developing spinal stabilization and the ability to resist rotation through the torso. Standing one-arm cable presses are far more useful as a core exercise than one to build your chest (Santana, Vera-Garcia, and McGill 2007). Pallof presses, standing one-arm cable presses, and other antirotation exercises are considerably more functional than many other core exercises. They're far more transferable to many activities you'll see in both sport and daily life.

Side Bends and Lateral-Flexion Exercises

Once popular, side bend variations have become less so in recent years. A lot of this is the result of a shift toward more core-focused and functional training approaches. Based on the function of the external obliques, there's no reason that exercises like these can't form part of a well-rounded abdominal training plan. Consider side bends for your obliques to be similar to crunches for your six-pack. If you want to target and strengthen your obliques, then side bend variations can be combined effectively with more rotational movements as well as exercises like pikes and rollouts that show high activation. Unfortunately, though, variations of side bends are often performed incorrectly. One common mistake is using a dumb-bell in each hand and simply laterally flexing from one side to the other. This is a waste of time and is highly ineffective. Chapter 9 will cover the most effective variations of these exercises and how to correct common technique flaws to get the most from them.

Loaded Carries

Heavy loaded carries such as farmer's walks and suitcase carries are effective exercises for activating your abdominal muscles while also teaching spinal stability. They can be used to teach abdominal bracing (taught throughout the exercise chapters) and the ability to resist lateral spine flexion and stability around the hip. They can achieve high activation levels in TVA and internal and external obliques. The greatest activation of these muscles is seen during the walking phase of the carry (McGill, McDermott, and Fenwick 2009). You should not simply stand still with a heavy weight in your hands and expect the same effect. Because of their applicability to daily and sporting activities, loaded carries are a highly functional exercise to train for these activities. Carries are also highly versatile, and while one variation can be used to further challenge your ability to resist lateral flexion, others can be used to activate your entire core or work other areas of your body. For both performance and aesthetics, loaded carries offer a good mix of both.

Explosive Medicine Ball and Battle Rope Exercises

Explosive exercises like those performed using battle ropes and medicine balls can offer fun and variety to your programming. The high velocity of these exercises makes them useful for athletes and helps prevent a loss of power as we age.

Preventing power loss is key for retaining muscle mass as we get older. So, while in the short term battle rope and medicine ball exercises offer an effective means to condition your abs and entire body, they're also an investment exercise for the future. Because of their explosive nature, they can show reasonable levels of muscle activation in your abdominal region, especially in the external obliques. To hit these areas even harder, you can use more chopping-type motions. Unilateral wave variations with ropes have also been shown to be effective (Calatayud 2015). It's worth noting, however, that despite respectable levels of peak muscle activation, overall muscle tension will be relatively low in these exercises because the duration of each repetition is relatively short. As an exercise to build muscle in the abdominal region, there are better options. Use explosive medicine ball slams and battle rope exercises for their host of other benefits instead.

Table 3.2 includes a summary of the types of exercises explained in this section along with the main use for the movements.

Table 3.2 Summary of Types of Exercise, Characteristics, and Potential Use in the Context of Abdominal Training

Exercise type	Example variations	Main movement	Plane of movement*	Main use
Crunch	Floor weighted Kneeling cable Stability ball	Spinal flexion	Moving in the sagittal plane	Rectus abdominis activation and hypertrophy
Sit-up	Floor body weight Eagle sit-up Hamstring activated	Spinal flexion Hip flexion	Moving in the sagittal plane	Rectus abdominis activation and hypertrophy
Reverse crunch and leg raise	Decline reverse crunch Garhammer raise Toes to bar	Spinal flexion Posterior pelvic tilt	Moving in the sagittal plane	Activation and hypertrophy of the rectus abdominis and obliques, particularly lower region
Pike and knee tuck	Stability ball Suspension trainer Core slider	Antiextension Posterior pelvic tilt Hip flexion	Resisting and moving in the sagittal plane	Activation and hypertrophy of all abdominal muscles; spinal stabilization
Rollout	Ab wheel Barbell Suspension fallout	Antiextension Spinal flexion Hip flexion	Resisting and moving in the sagittal plane	Activation and hypertrophy of all abdominal muscles; spinal stabilization
Body saw	Feet walking Suspension Core slider	Antiextension	Resisting in the sagittal plane	Activation and hypertrophy of all abdominal muscles; spinal stabilization
Twisting crunch and twisting sit-up	Russian twist Body-weight oblique crunch Kneeling cable side crunch	Spinal flexion Spinal rotation	Movement in transverse and sagittal planes	May be useful for activation and hypertrophy of obliques

(continued)

Table 3.2 (continued)

Exercise type	Example variations	Main movement	Plane of movement*	Main use
Chopping exercises	Cable chop Band chop Landmine rotation	Spinal rotation Hip extension	Movement in the transverse plane	Functional and performance-based exercise; activation of the obliques
Front plank progression	Weighted Long-lever PPT Suspension	Antiextension	Resisting in the sagittal plane	May be useful for overall abdominal and core activation; need to be progressed
Bird dog and dead bug	Floor body weight Dead-bug pullover Bird-dog row	Antirotation	Resisting in the transverse plane	May be useful for overall abdominal and core activation; need to be progressed
Pallof press and similar	Standing cable Pallof Supine Pallof Suspension Pallof	Antirotation	Resisting in the transverse and frontal plane	May be useful for overall abdominal and core activation; need to be progressed
Side bend and similar	Cable side bend Tate side bend Side plank crunch	Lateral spine flexion	Movement in the frontal plane	Training the external obliques in relative isolation
Loaded carry	Farmer's Suitcase Waiter	Total body	Multiplane	Functional and performance-based exercise; activation of the entire core
Explosive rope and medicine ball exercises	Battle rope chop Rotational medicine ball slam Heavy battle rope or ball slam	Total body	Multiplane	Functional and performance-based exercise; explosiveness and conditioning

*Sagittal plane: Divides the body laterally into right and left halves.
Transverse plane: Divides the body into upper and lower halves.
Frontal plane: Divides the body anteriorly and posteriorly into front and back halves.

SUMMARY

Many people use the terms *core* and *abs* interchangeably, which causes confusion when training and targeting either. While core training should be used to pursue spinal and pelvic stability, abdominal training is the targeting of four very specific muscles for aesthetic purposes: the rectus abdominis, transverse abdominis, internal obliques, and external obliques. Some exercises are more core focused, while others very much isolate your abdominals. Many exercises overlap and can be effective for training both your core and abdominals. Blending these approaches produces the most impressive results and is a continuing theme throughout this book. In the next chapter, we'll take a look at how cardio-based exercise can be added for even greater progress.

Using Cardio as a Tool

We've all heard the saying that "abs are built in the kitchen." Now, unless your kitchen also doubles as your exercise area, then this just isn't true. It's more accurate to say that "abs are built with resistance, carved in the kitchen, and cut up with cardio." But this doesn't have the same ring to it, does it?

Subjecting your abs to resistance training is essential for them to become more dense, with more deeply etched lines. The exercises listed in part II alongside the principles you learned in chapter 1 will allow you to develop your abs. But to see what you've built, you also need a low level of body fat so nothing is hiding it. The optimal percentage of body fat varies depending on where you store it and the measurement methods you use (see chapter 5). Generally speaking for most men, visible abs start to appear at 10 to 14 percent body fat. For a completely chiseled look no matter what lighting you're in, it's closer to 5 to 9 percent body fat.

For women looking to get in great shape, 15 to 19 percent body fat will provide good definition in the abdominals and obliques. A body fat percentage of 10 to 14 percent is as low as most women want to go and still display deeply etched abdominals. If you're not anywhere near these figures right now, then creating a slight calorie deficit will enable you to lose the body fat covering your abdominals.

In this chapter, you'll learn how to use cardiovascular exercise as a tool to assist in revealing your abs. Although it's not within the scope of this book to discuss dietary requirements, you'll also find simple nutrition principles that will help you along the way.

ENERGY BALANCE AND FAT LOSS

When we speak of energy balance, we're simply talking about energy input and energy output. The most common way this is described is as calories consumed and calories burned. The difference between the two (input versus output) determines whether excess energy is stored or lost. Your body stores this excess and unburned energy in a few ways; however, for the purpose of keeping it simple and on point, unused energy (calories) usually show up as the extra layer of fat between your abdominals and what you see in the mirror.

If you gain body weight, then by definition your energy input was greater than your output. If you lose weight, then your energy input was less than your output. And, if your weight remains the same, your input and output were balanced. Things such as digestion and water retention can cause fluctuations in body weight, but generally this is how energy balance affects body weight. You should also keep in mind that weight gain or weight loss does not necessarily mean *fat* gain or fat loss. The difference between the two and how to achieve weight loss in the form of fat rather than muscle is referenced throughout this chapter.

Energy Output

We typically describe energy input as the total calories you consume daily. On the other hand, the way we describe energy output is in terms of your total daily energy expenditure (TDEE; see figure 4.1). Your TDEE is made up of the following (Trexler, Smith-Ryan, and Norton 2014):

- *Exercise activity thermogenesis (EAT):* The energy used in purposeful exercise activities—for example, resistance training and cardiovascular exercise. EAT makes up approximately 5 percent of TDEE. However, for people regularly participating in purposeful exercise activity, it's believed to account for up to 15 to 30 percent (Von Loeffelholz and Birkenfeld 2018).

- *Thermic effect of food (TEF):* The energy used in digestion and absorption of food energy. This varies according to the types of foods you eat, among other factors. This makes up approximately 10 percent of TDEE.

- *Nonexercise activity thermogenesis (NEAT):* The energy used in activities other than sleeping, eating, and exercise—for example, the energy burned during daily activities such as walking, gardening, cooking, and cleaning. NEAT makes up 15 percent of your TDEE.

- *Basal metabolic rate (BMR):* The number of calories your body needs to function. This accounts for roughly 70 percent of your TDEE.

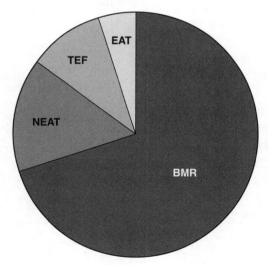

Components of total daily energy expenditure

Figure 4.1 Components of total daily energy expenditure (TDEE). BMR=basal metabolic rate (70%); NEAT=nonexercise activity thermogenesis (15%); TEF=thermic effect of food (10%); EAT=exercise activity thermogenesis (5%).

A few options are available for increasing TDEE (energy output). While we do not have much control over BMR daily, we do have the ability to increase energy output by increasing the following:

- *NEAT*: This can be achieved by being more active in general throughout each day, including getting your steps in and maybe making an excuse to trim the lawn or tidy the house more often. It's also a good excuse to wash your car by hand rather than take it to the local drive-through car wash.
- *TEF*: This can be achieved by eating the right foods. For example, it's been understood for a long time that protein requires more energy to digest and has a higher thermic effect than fat and carbohydrate (Glickman et al. 1948). A diet higher in protein is therefore beneficial for augmenting fat loss.
- *EAT*: This is achieved by increasing energy output through resistance exercise and cardiovascular activities. This book has you covered on both these fronts.

Where Cardio Fits In

Cardio training is not essential to creating a calorie deficit. Providing your TDEE exceeds the amount of energy (calories) you put into your body, you will lose weight. Weight loss and fat loss are not the same thing, though. If your goal is to make radical changes in your body composition, you will achieve more muscle gain and fat loss if your calorie intake remains high while your output is also high. This means consuming more calories but also boosting your energy output, largely through resistance exercise and cardio activities. For example, you will get better results if you burn an extra 200 calories per day with exercise and are allowed to eat an extra 200 calories instead of forgoing the 200 calories and not exercising as much. This is a far better strategy for most people because it enables them to create a slight deficit while avoiding overtraining and muscle wasting. Cardio is one of the most effective tools for increasing energy output through EAT. If you have fat to lose, then a good cardio program coupled with nutritional strategies will work alongside your targeted ab workouts in attaining a lean and athletic-looking midsection.

TOP FIVE NUTRITION TIPS FOR REVEALING YOUR SIX-PACK

Our energy intake is controlled by the amount of food we eat. In conjunction with an increased energy output through exercise and activity, eating the right amount of food can help you create a calorie deficit that will reveal six-pack abs. Here are the top tips to lead you in the right direction. For more information on this topic, pick up one of the many Human Kinetics books that cover diets for aesthetics and performance in more detail.

1. *All good fat-loss diets share this common theme.* If you have a layer of fat covering your abs, then no matter how hard you train them or how closely you follow the guidelines in this book, you'll never be able to see them. If you want to see your abs, then you need to lose the fat. And to lose body fat, you need to be in a slight caloric deficit. No matter what nutritional approach you use or diet plan you follow, all plans that work do so only because they place you in a caloric deficit. Cutting out certain food groups (e.g., gluten, wheat, dairy) work for some

people because they eliminate calories; intermittent fasting can work if it means limiting calories to a certain eating window (less than you were eating before); eating less processed food and more vegetables will result in eating fewer calories while feeling more full; cutting carbohydrate or fat from your diet just cuts out calories, too. The best diet for rapid changes to your physique is the one you can stick to and will allow you to eat the right amount of food to fuel your progress.

2. *You can only manage what you can monitor.* Your macronutrients, or macros, are protein (4 calories per gram), fat (9 calories per gram), and carbohydrate (4 calories per gram). Alcohol is also a macronutrient at 7 calories per gram. The total of these macronutrients makes up your total daily calories. For example, if you eat 25 grams of protein, you have consumed 100 calories, 25 grams of carbohydrate also equates to 100 calories, and 25 grams of fat equates to 225 calories. To manage your macronutrients and calories, you either need massive awareness of what you're eating or you need to track your food intake. For even the most experienced person, the latter is the safest bet, and there are mobile phone apps that make this easy. If you don't monitor your food intake, then you won't know whether you're consuming the right number of calories to fuel your workouts while enabling yourself to lose fat at the same time. If you monitor it, then you can manage it!

3. *It doesn't matter whether you choose low fat or low carb.* There's nothing inherently special about reducing either your fats or carbohydrates other than the fact that limiting either of these will reduce your overall calorie intake. Because you want to maintain a high protein intake throughout a fat loss phase (maintaining a caloric deficit for a period of time), you need to reduce either your fat or carbohydrate calories or both. Most people achieve the most impressive and sustainable physique when carbohydrate remains in the diet. Especially when tracking foods, allowing carbohydrate in your diet while reducing fat a little offers the most flexibility. Let's assume that you're preparing for a physique competition or photo shoot. Carbohydrate allows your training quality to remain high and your muscles to feel full. However, a reduced-carbohydrate diet *can* work if you prefer to eat more fat and limit your carbohydrate. What works and what is optimal are different things, though, and long-term sustainability of any diet type is key.

4. *See calorie totals as weekly, not daily, goals.* We've all been here: You start your training and diet overhaul on Monday, and then over the weekend you end up exceeding your calorie goal. It might have been planned or just a spur-of-the-moment thing. And there's no problem with that; you deserve a life after all. But now your weekly calorie count no longer averages the 2,000 per day you determined would put you in a slight deficit. One 4,000-calorie day just made your daily average 2,285 calories! There's nothing wrong with having a higher-calorie or planned cheat day each week, but factor that into your weekly average.

5. *Stay accountable.* There's a reason why experienced physique athletes and even professional coaches have their own coaches. Having someone to keep you accountable and on track is a big advantage on any journey. The help of a professional is invaluable in ensuring you get the results you deserve and that all your diet and exercise efforts are directed in the right way. If getting professional support isn't your thing, using a "buddy-up" system is another way to keep you on track. All you need is a friend or family member who wants to undergo the same transformation you do, and then you can be there to support each other along the

way. You might both work through this book, for example, and do weekly check-ins to track how each of you is progressing. Chapter 5 will show you what you can monitor along the way to know whether you're progressing in the right direction.

THE BEST CARDIO TO LOOK GREAT NAKED

Adding cardiovascular exercise to your weekly routine will increase energy output, making it easier for you to achieve a slight caloric deficit. It'll allow you to lose any fat covering your abdominals without having to restrict your calorie intake as much. But, before you get carried away and start amassing hours of cardio exercise each week, you should know a few things to get the best results from a physique standpoint.

To optimize body composition (fat loss and muscle gain), you need to do the right amount of cardio at the right intensity. This will vary depending on several factors, including your own training psychology. Keep in mind that you're not concerned with enhancing performance here or developing specific energy systems. Instead, the cardio you do will have the sole intent of helping you look great with your shirt off. We are therefore most concerned with the calorie burn, recoverability, and muscle-sparing ability of certain cardio workouts.

It's generally understood that four forms of exercise fall into the cardio category. To understand these forms of cardio you also need a basic understanding of how oxygen is (or isn't) used during exercise.

Exercise and Oxygen Consumption

$\dot{V}O_2$max is the highest rate of oxygen consumption attainable during maximal or exhaustive exercise. As exercise intensity increases, so does oxygen consumption until you reach the point where the amount of oxygen your body consumes plateaus, even as exercise intensity continues to increase. At this point, exercise switches from aerobic (with oxygen) to anaerobic (without oxygen).

Supramaximal Interval Training (SMIT)

Supramaximal interval training typically involves interspersing extremely high-intensity periods of exercise (above 100 percent of $\dot{V}O_2$max) with passive (fully resting) or active (low-intensity) periods. SMIT workouts produce the highest energy output (calorie burn) in a given amount of time but are also shorter and harder to recover from.

High-Intensity Interval Training (HIIT)

HIIT involves interspersing high-intensity periods of exercise, performed at or close to 100 percent of your $\dot{V}O_2$max, with periods of passive recovery or active recovery. HIIT workouts are relatively short and are suggested to be more muscle sparing than lower-intensity workouts. But they are harder to perform mentally, recovery from them is slow, and you can't perform them as frequently as you might like. For these reasons, physique athletes usually don't prepare for a competition or photo shoot using large amounts of SMIT and HIIT. Although technically a more efficient workout to get you shredded fast, recovery aspects as well as psychological factors should be considered when undergoing a body transformation process.

Steady-State Cardio Training

Steady-state training is a standard bout of longer-duration aerobic exercise, typically performed for 30 minutes or more. It can include running or be performed on equipment such as an exercise bike or elliptical trainer. Some people have proposed that these workouts are muscle wasting. But research shows otherwise, and it may even *enhance* gains in untrained men (Mikkola et al. 2012). How effective or detrimental this form of exercise is varies from person to person, and will also be dependent on the other forms and volumes of training being done at the same time. The correct balance between cardiovascular and resistance work is important. Too much cardiovascular exercise will slow your progress in gaining size and strength. While cardio will help you strip the fat that covers your abdominals, too much cardio work can make it difficult for your abs to recover and grow from their targeted workouts.

Metabolic Conditioning Protocols (MCPs)

MCPs are a mixture of conditioning and strength work. They require moving heavy implements (e.g., weights, tires, ropes, push sled) fast or for long periods of time. They're the ideal training tool for athletes who need power and strength endurance and for those who just get bored with regular cardio workouts. When using MCPs for cardio exercise, a 1:1 to 1:2 work-to-rest ratio is recommended for fat loss. Other protocols focus on improving performance outcomes.

SPECIFICITY OF CARDIO TRAINING

Chapter 1 introduced the principle of specificity. This principle applies to both cardio and resistance training. For sport athletes, specificity might mean matching the work-to-rest ratios within their sport to their cardio activities. For example, the average work-to-rest ratio during a National Football League drive is about 1:6 (about 5 seconds of work and 30 seconds of rest) (Mikkola et al. 2012). So, if you are a football player, your cardio workout might use a 1:6 work-to-rest ratio in order to mimic that. Specificity for you right now is dictated by your goals. And, as we discussed in chapter 1, the goal is to build muscle and burn body fat. Specificity in your cardio workouts is determined by what will help you burn fat the fastest while retaining muscle.

WHICH TYPE OF CARDIO IS RIGHT FOR ME?

To develop a chiseled set of core muscles, they need to grow and get stronger just like any other muscle. Because of certain hormonal and biochemical reactions triggered by most forms of cardiovascular exercise, adaptations resulting from the cardio work will interfere with your muscle and strength development. Plus, the more cardio you do, the more efficient your body becomes at doing it, which causes you to burn fewer calories. When you are training for a specific goal, always remember the SAID (specific adaptation to imposed demands) principle. Your body will always specifically adapt to the demands you place on it, and it doesn't care whether that gives you a six-pack or not. Your body is clever like that, but it's frustrating for you if you're forgetting to send it clear messages.

If you want to burn calories and body fat, higher-intensity methods tend to be more muscle sparing and time efficient. Weight circuits, metabolic resistance training, and even Tabata or half-Tabata intervals are good options. However, many athletes don't do well with these forms of training when they are running low on calories while trying to optimize fat loss. They might plan to do a SMIT or HIIT workout, but when faced with it, the motivation and intensity are too low to be productive. Additionally, the high-impact and intense nature of these workouts can hinder recovery and affect the targeted resistance workouts.

On paper, higher-intensity and metabolic conditioning workouts are more effective and save time, making them a far more appealing prospect than sitting on an exercise bike for 30 to 40 minutes. However, you might find aerobic workouts more appealing and sustainable. And they won't kill your progress as long as you don't overdo it, and you choose low-impact methods such as cycling, uphill walking, and swimming. These will help you burn calories and affect your resistance workouts less than higher-impact aerobic workouts such as running on the road. Drawing from anecdotal experience, I've seen many people get into great shape by managing their calorie input, doing their resistance workouts, and simply going for brisk daily walks.

When choosing the forms of cardio you want to do each week, consider the following:

- What forms of cardio do you enjoy most?
- What forms of cardio are you most likely to stick with even when your energy levels are low?
- Which of these will help you burn the most calories in the shortest amount of time?

There is no rule for the number of extra calories you should burn through cardio each week. It would be smart, however, to factor in at least two or three cardio workouts each week for general health. Be sure to factor in the calories burned during cardio workouts when setting your goals for calorie input (see table 4.1).

Table 4.1 Energy Expenditure in Physical Activities

	Calories used per hour based on weight				
	100 lb (45 kg)	**120 lb (54 kg)**	**150 lb (68 kg)**	**180 lb (82 kg)**	**200 lb (91 kg)**
Backpacking or hiking	307	348	410	472	513
Badminton	255	289	340	391	425
Baseball	210	238	280	322	350
Basketball (half-court)	225	240	300	345	375
Bicycling (normal speed)	157	178	210	242	263
Bowling	155	176	208	240	261
Canoeing (4 mph [6.5 kph])	276	344	414	504	558
Circuit training	247	280	330	380	413
Dance (ballet/modern)	240	300	360	432	480
Dance (aerobic)	300	360	450	540	600
Dance (social)	174	222	264	318	348
Fitness calisthenics	232	263	310	357	388

(continued)

Table 4.1 *(continued)*

	Calories used per hour based on weight				
	100 lb (45 kg)	120 lb (54 kg)	150 lb (68 kg)	180 lb (82 kg)	200 lb (91 kg)
Football	225	255	300	345	375
Golf (walking)	187	212	250	288	313
Gymnastics	232	263	310	357	388
Horseback riding	180	204	240	276	300
Interval training	487	552	650	748	833
Jogging (5.5 mph [9 kph])	487	552	650	748	833
Judo or karate	232	263	310	357	388
Jumping rope (continuous)	525	595	700	805	875
Racquetball or handball	450	510	600	690	750
Running (10 mph [16 kph])	625	765	900	1,035	1,125
Skating (ice or roller)	262	297	350	403	438
Skiing (cross-country)	525	595	700	805	875
Skiing (downhill)	450	510	600	690	750
Soccer	405	459	540	575	621
Softball (fastpitch)	210	238	280	322	350
Swimming (slow laps)	240	272	320	368	400
Swimming (fast laps)	420	530	630	768	846
Tennis	315	357	420	483	525
Volleyball	262	297	350	403	483
Walking	204	258	318	372	426
Weight training	352	399	470	541	558

Reprinted by permission from C.B. Corbin, D.M. Castelli, B.A. Sibley, and G.C. Le Masurier, *Fitness for Life,* 7th ed. (Champaign, IL: Human Kinetics, 2022), 355.

TOP SIX WAYS TO KEEP CARDIO INTERESTING

Cardio doesn't have to be boring. And you don't always need to do separate cardio sessions to burn a few extra calories. If you don't have the time to do separate cardio sessions, then adding shorter "finishers" to the end of your workouts is an efficient way to get it done. Here are simple cardio finishers that will help you keep it interesting:

1. *Master the jump rope.* Skipping with a rope is one of the simplest and best forms of total-body conditioning out there. It will injury proof your ankles and knees, it's lower impact and easier to recover from than running, and it requires very little equipment or space. Try dusting off your skipping rope at the end of your ab workouts for a fun way to condition and burn a few extra calories. Set a timer for three to five minutes and see what you can get done.

2. *Get athletic with agility drills.* These drills are typically used by athletes and sport coaches to develop agility and change-of-direction speed. However, you can also turn them into cardiovascular conditioning exercises. Hill and shuttle sprints can be effective, but changing directions, turning, and cutting are a whole lot more interesting. Plus they will get your heart rate up much sooner. For fat loss, try using agility drills as intervals with a 1:1 to 1:2 work-to-rest ratio. That is, if you set up a drill that takes you 20 seconds to complete, take 20 to 40 seconds to rest. T-drills and zigzag and Union Jack drills are simple to set up with just a handful of cones (see figure 4.2).

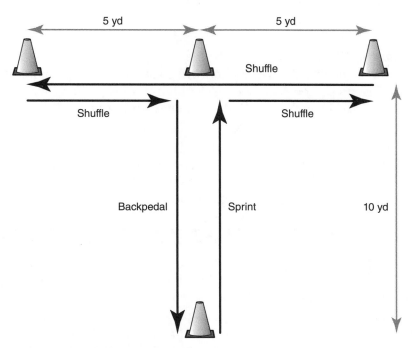

Figure 4.2 Example of a T agility drill.

3. *Longer-duration loaded carries.* Grab something heavy and walk with pride and purpose. In chapter 10, you'll find a description of the one-arm farmer's carry you can try. You can also perform a basic farmer's carry holding weight in both hands instead of just one, as shown in drill 5 later in this chapter. This has less of a core component to it, but is more taxing for your entire muscular and cardiovascular systems. You have many options for loaded carries; all you need is weight (e.g., dumbbells, kettlebells, sandbag, trap bar) and space to walk. For fat loss, 60 to 90 seconds walking followed by 60 to 90 seconds resting works well. Try four to six sets to warm up or finish your ab workouts.

4. *Metabolic resistance training (MRT).* In short, MRT is a form of circuit training that uses the same resistance throughout (sometimes called a *complex*). You pick up a weight (e.g., barbell, dumbbell, kettlebell) and do four to six exercises without stopping for a complete set (see table 4.2). Because of its specific structure, you won't underload some movements while overloading others as typically happens during most other styles of circuit training.

Table 4.2 Sample Metabolic Resistance Training (MRT) Circuit Using Dumbbells or Kettlebells*

Exercise	Reps	Weight	Rest
1a: Reverse lunge	6-8	Start with a weight you can lunge 10 times on each leg	15 sec, straight to 1b
1b: Bent-over row	6-8	Same weight as previous	15 sec, straight to 1c
1c: Overhead push press	6-8	Same weight as previous	15 sec, straight to 1d
1d: Romanian deadlift	6-8	Same weight as previous	120 sec, return to 1a; repeat × 3-5 rounds

*Repeat the circuit three to five times.

5. *Ladder drills.* Low-intensity plyometric drills are a fun way to finish off a workout, get your heart rate up, and improve coordination. Try combining ladder drills with a Tabata protocol (20 seconds of high-intensity efforts with 10 seconds of passive recovery for eight rounds) to mix up your cardio sessions.

6. *Cycle or walk and learn.* It's low impact and easy to recover from and you can listen to audiobooks or podcasts while doing it. It's not a finisher in the same sense as the other exercises, but if you prefer to finish your resistance workouts with low-intensity cardio, then cycling or incline walking are the best options that allow you to do other things at the same time.

TEN CARDIO EXERCISES YOU SHOULD KNOW

Cardio exercise is just one tool you have at your disposal to increase energy output. If your energy (calorie) output is slightly greater than your input (i.e., your TDEE is greater than the calories you consume), then you will lose body fat. This needs to be managed carefully though, because if your energy deficit is too great, then you risk losing muscle and strength. One approach that works very well for simultaneous fat loss and muscle gain is to determine your maintenance level of calories (i.e., the calorie intake that allows your weight to remain stable for at least a week or two), and then create a very slight deficit by adding cardio exercise on top of that. For example, if your maintenance calories were 2,500 per day, then you could keep your exercise (EAT) and NEAT activities the same and eat 250 calories less (a mild deficit). Or you could eat the same 2,500 calories and burn an additional 250 calories each day through EAT and NEAT (still, a small deficit). The latter method will achieve far superior changes in body composition while improving health markers at the same time. The following exercises are the most useful ways to perform your cardio.

1
SHUTTLE RUN

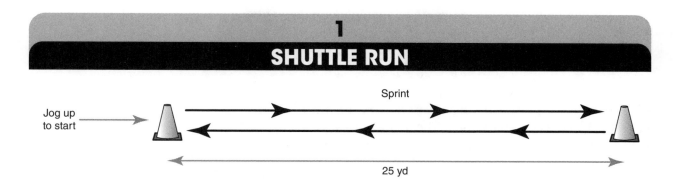

Shuttle runs are old-school drills that have stood the test of time. They might well give you flashbacks to high school physical education classes or punishers on the school sports field, but they're useful for your six-pack workouts. They're a good way to incorporate SMIT and HIIT workouts into your weekly training and require no equipment. Just don't start thinking you're in the Olympic 100-meter finals. Start with 60 to 70 percent speed efforts and focus on technique.

Setup

- Place two cones 25 yards (23 m) apart.
- You can also use water bottles or whatever is available.

Performance

1. Jog up to the starting cone, and then sprint all the way to the final cone.
2. Touch the cone, turn, and sprint back.
3. Repeat 25-yard sprints between the two cones for as many times as you need to achieve your target distance.
4. A total of 100 to 300 yards (90 to 274 m) work well for fat loss.
5. Between each shuttle run rest two to three times as long as you ran. For example, if the shuttles took you 30 seconds to complete, then rest 60 to 90 seconds before repeating.

Tips for Success

- Do rolling starts by jogging up to your first cone before sprinting the rest of the way. This will limit the chance of your hamstrings suddenly giving out midshuttle.
- Anticipate the finish cone and focus on proper deceleration mechanics.

2
AGILITY RUN

No rule states that you have to run in a straight line to burn body fat. Agility runs have you moving forward, backward, sideways, spinning, and cutting your way to shredded abs. You have plenty of agility drills to choose from. Here's how to do a simple zigzag drill.

Setup

- Place cones in a zigzag pattern, using the spacing of your choice.
- You can space the cones randomly to mix it up.

Performance

1. Slalom through the cones, going around the outside of each one.
2. The closer the cones, the sharper you'll have to step.
3. Do this as quickly as possible, and then walk back to the start.
4. For fat loss, do this as many times as you can for 60 seconds, and then rest for 60 to 90 seconds before repeating for up to five rounds.
5. Vary this drill by stepping on the inside of the cones and bending down to touch each one.

Tips for Success

- Keep the drills simple to start and focus on proper acceleration, deceleration, and change-of-direction mechanics.
- Start with softer rather than sharper turns, especially if it's been some time since you've had to sidestep a cone (or person).

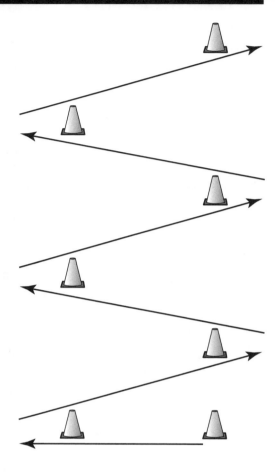

3
BASIC SLED PUSH

Basic sled pushes are a high-intensity cardio exercise that have a reputation for being a real leg and lung burner. They're a great full-body conditioning workout, and with the number of ways you can use a push sled, you'll never get bored. As far as high-intensity training methods go, sled pushes are relatively low impact and joint friendly. If your gym has a sled, you should make the most of it.

Setup

- Grip the handles of the sled. This can vary depending on sled design.
- Place one foot in front, with your knee and hip flexed.
- Place the other foot back, with your hip and knee fully extended.

Performance

1. Stay low, keep a flat back, and drive your legs hard to push the sled as fast as you can.
2. You may also add weight and move the sled at a slower pace.
3. For fat loss, start with 60 to 90 seconds of pushing, with 60 to 90 seconds of active or passive recovery.
4. Repeat for four to six rounds.

Tips for Success

- Drag the sled as an alternative.
- Add a suspension trainer or Olympic rings to your sled so you can backpedal, step sideways, and move in other creative ways to condition your heart and lungs while burning body fat.

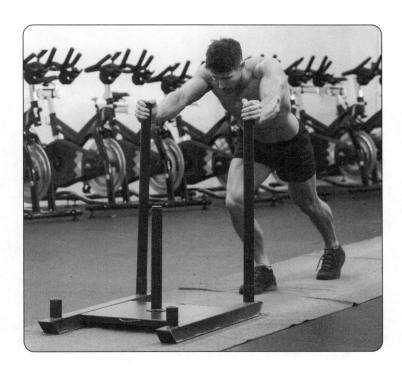

4

BATTLE ROPES

Battle ropes are all the rage in HIIT workouts and for good reason. Unlike most forms of cardio, this is more upper-body focused and offers beginners a relatively simple way to increase calorie output. Start with an alternating-waves pattern and then get creative.

Setup

Begin with the ropes in hand, pulling slightly to create enough tension in the ropes that you have to resist.

Performance

1. Grab the ropes, slightly bend your knees, and then alternate your arms up and down to create waves in the ropes.
2. Flutter the ropes aggressively and try to maintain the same effort for the duration of the set.
3. Start with 20 to 30 seconds of work, with 40 to 60 seconds of rest for five rounds.
4. Adjust your work-to-rest ratios and the thickness of the ropes as your fitness levels improve.

Tips for Success

- As a simple addition to the alternating-waves pattern, try reverse lunging, sideways lunging, or squatting at the same time.
- Other patterns include creating both waves at the same time, rope slams, sideways waves, uppercuts, and air punches.

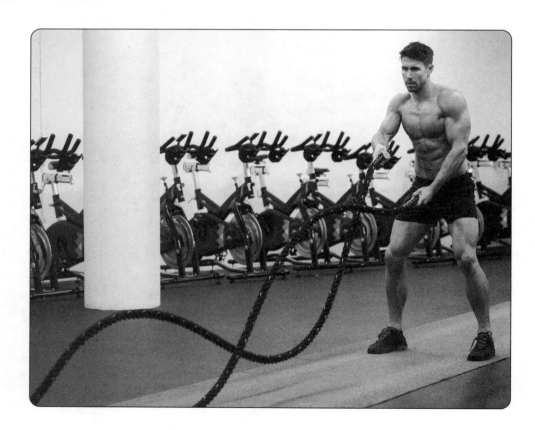

5
BASIC FARMER'S CARRY

The basic farmer's carry is either a core exercise or a cardio exercise depending on the protocols you use. That makes these a useful addition to your fat-loss training and general conditioning when developing your abs.

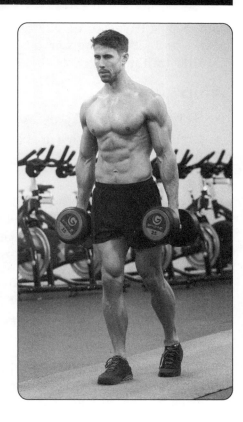

Setup

- Hold dumbbells or kettlebells by your sides.
- Keep a tight grip, stay tall, and keep your shoulders back.

Performance

1. Go for a walk.
2. Walk proud and with purpose.
3. Keep your core braced. Imagine 360 degrees of air around your spine and with your abdominals contracted.
4. Walk in a straight line and then back again for 60 to 90 seconds. Rest for 60 to 90 seconds.
5. Repeat for six rounds.

Tips for Success

Variations are to walk in a figure-8 and forward and backward. You can carry different implements by your sides and also carry them in front or overhead.

6
ROWING MACHINE

Many people have a love–hate relationship with the rower, but those who enjoy it can get a great calorie- and fat-burning workout from it. The rower can be used for steady-state as well as SMIT and HIIT training protocols.

Setup

- Sit on the rower and strap your feet in.
- Grab the handle with a double-overhand grip.
- Begin with your torso upright and a slight flex in your knees.

Performance

1. Drive your legs and hips and pull as hard as you can.
2. Each action should be coordinated like a "whip" from your legs to hips to arms.
3. This is best done for intervals of 20 to 40 seconds of all-out effort followed by 20 to 40 seconds of recovery.
4. You may also use the rowing machine for steady-state cardio training, maintaining a moderate effort level for 20 minutes or more (4 or 5 out of 10 in terms of effort).

Tips for Success

- When performing intervals, an active rather than passive recovery is usually best. Some rowers automatically switch off if they don't move for even short periods of time. Keep your legs and arms moving with an easy row between harder intervals.
- Choose a resistance that best suits you. Longer-duration rowing will require a lower resistance, while higher-intensity efforts require a higher resistance.

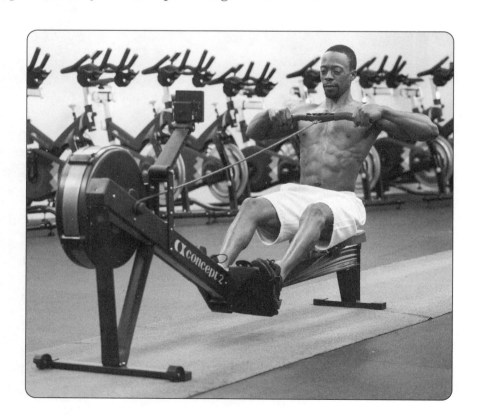

7
TREADMILL

Nothing beats a walk outside in the fresh air and sunshine. It's the best way to get your daily vitamin D while watching the world go by. But if a treadmill is your only option or you just prefer it, then using it can be just as effective. You can perform speed intervals, aerobic runs, and incline and brisk walking on it.

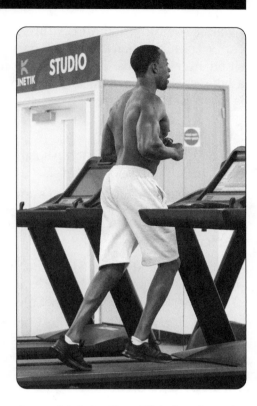

Setup

Set the treadmill to a speed and incline that suits you.

Performance

1. Begin running or walking at a pace that matches the treadmill speed.
2. Move your arms at a pace that matches your legs. If you're running or sprinting, then drive your arms hard to match the speed of your legs.
3. If you're walking on an incline, do not hold the handles in front unless you absolutely need to. Use your arms and stop cheating.

Tips for Success

Don't underestimate walking on a treadmill at a brisk pace and on a high incline. This is a favorite among high-level physique athletes for good reason.

8
CYCLING, SPINNING, AND AIR BIKE

Cycling, spinning, and Air Bike are excellent forms of cardio training when fat loss and overall body composition are your goals. The low-impact nature of using a bike causes little wear and tear to your body and is a relatively easy form of exercise to recover from.

Setup

- Set the saddle to about hip height and the handlebars to a comfortable level.
- Set your resistance to what's appropriate according to the type of cardio you're performing.

Performance

1. For SMIT and HIIT, pedal fast or with a high resistance for short periods. For example, 30 seconds of effort, with 30 seconds of recovery riding.
2. For steady-state training, work at a moderate effort (4 or 5 out of 10 in terms of effort) for a longer duration, say 30 minutes or more.

Tips for Success

- If you have a spinning bike, then you can mix it up with some peddling in the saddle and some out of it.
- A bike is well suited for recovery-based sessions that enhance the results of the rest of your training. It's fine to go easy sometimes.

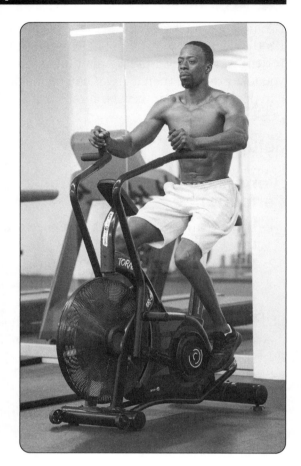

9
ELLIPTICAL TRAINER

The elliptical trainer is a piece of equipment readily available in most gyms and, much like cycling, can offer a low-impact form of training suitable for most people.

Setup

Step on the elliptical trainer and grab the upright handles.

Performance

1. Pump your legs and arms and stay tall as you perform the action.
2. Both your arms and legs should have equal input.
3. Use a moderate intensity (4 or 5 out of 10 in terms of effort) for 20 to 30 minutes.

Tips for Success

- Cardio exercise on machines doesn't have to be limited to one piece of equipment.
- If you're using steady-state cardio, try doing half on one machine, and then half on another. For example, do 15 minutes on an elliptical trainer and then 15 minutes on a bike.

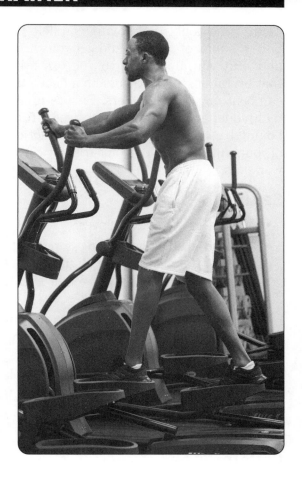

10
BOXING BAG

There is no doubt that boxing can help you burn a bunch of calories and get you shredded. But you also need to keep in mind that brutal boxing workouts on a heavy bag can beat up your shoulders. Ensure proper technique, and even look into water-filled boxing bags to take some of the impact out of your punches for more joint-friendly cardio workouts.

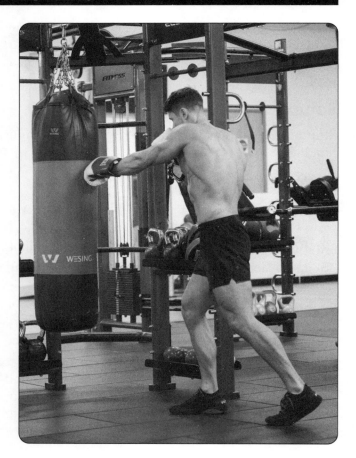

Setup

- You'll need a bag and gloves.
- Assume an effective fighting stance, with your feet staggered and slightly wider than your hips and your weight evenly distributed.
- Keep a small amount of tension in your abdominals throughout.
- Your rear elbow and forearm stay close to your body, while your lead elbow is slightly in front of your body.
- Your head should be slightly tilted forward and "glued" to your collar bone.

Performance

1. In the fighting stance as described, perform a combination of jabs, punches, uppercuts, and hooks. You may also kick the bag if it's suitable.
2. Stay light on your toes and "float" around the bag.
3. Perform two- or three-minute rounds with one to two minutes of rest between each.

Tips for Success

- Seek a knowledgeable boxing coach to ensure your technique is both safe and effective.
- Water-filled boxing bags are worth seeking out. They cause less impact on your joints (especially your wrists), making them a better cardio choice than a heavy bag.

Chapter 5

Four Ways to Track Your Six-Pack Progress

In chapter 4, we discussed the importance of having levels of body fat low enough that your abdominals are visible and how cardio training can help create a caloric deficit that will lead to a leaner physique. Generally speaking, a good body fat target for visible abs is 10 to 14 percent in men and 15 to 19 percent in women. For a completely chiseled look, it should be 5 to 9 percent in men and 10 to 14 percent in women. In this chapter, we briefly discuss the best way to measure your progress based on common assessment methods. We then summarize how best to use this information to determine which program to use and the one thing you can do right now that will greatly increase your chances of achieving your ideal physique.

WHY MEASURE BODY FAT?

To see your abs, you need to reach body fat levels low enough to reveal what's underneath. A body fat percentage of 10 to 14 in men allows you to see good definition and lines starting to appear around the abdominals and obliques. This can vary, of course, depending on where you store most of your body fat, but at around 12 percent body fat, most men will start to see a vertical line appear down the middle of their abdominal area. This is the *linea alba* (Latin for *white line*). This happens for most women at about 15 percent body fat.

How much you lower your body fat percentage depends on the look you're going for and how deeply etched you want your abs to be. The lower you store your body fat, the more difficult these extremes are to achieve and maintain. If you prefer the truly "ripped" look that comes with extremely low levels of body fat, know that the reality for most people is that this rarely can be maintained for more than a few weeks or even just a single photo shoot or competition. Whatever your goals and how far you want to take it, you need to monitor how close you are to these ultimate targets and compare them to where you are right now. You also need to know whether you're staying on track. As stated in the previous chapter, what you can monitor, you can manage!

Tracking changes in lean mass (mass that isn't body fat) is of particular use because these numbers can represent gains or losses in muscle mass. When trying to optimally grow muscle and build your abs, you want to see your lean mass increase while maintaining your body fat level. On the other hand, if you're trying to optimize fat loss to reveal the abs you've built, then you want to see your body fat go down while you maintain muscle mass. As is common with many other training and dieting approaches that place you in a caloric deficit, losing fat without losing muscle can be a struggle. The programs in this book will help you achieve this balance, but it's important to monitor your changes so you can make adjustments when necessary.

If you're going for extremes, such as preparing for a physique photo shoot or competition, you can use methods to assess how flat or full your muscles look. This can determine whether you need to alter your nutritional strategy so you can bring your best look to the photography studio or to the competition stage. The art and science of competition and photo shoot preparation are outside the scope of this book, but the methods you will use to monitor changes in your physique will be the same.

There are a variety of ways to assess body composition. Dual-energy X-ray absorptiometry (DEXA) scans and air displacement plethysmography using Bod Pods require equipment found in a lab. However, we are concerned with more practical and accessible forms of assessment. The aforementioned methods are considered the gold-standard in measurement techniques, but you need access to techniques that can be used weekly without costing much time or money. That being said, paying for access to a DEXA scan or Bod Pod once or twice a year will give you useful feedback in the long term.

This chapter describes practical and accessible tools that cost very little (if anything) and techniques that can be used once per week without taking more than a few minutes of your time. These are practices a coach might ask you to use as a check-in as you go through a body transformation process, or things you should assess yourself during more intensive phases of training and dieting. If you want abs fast, then you need to familiarize yourself with one (or a few) of the following techniques.

BODY FAT SCALES

These are the scales you commonly find at your gym or already have in your bathroom. Quite often these have a function that allows you to measure body composition: your fat and muscle makeup. Many manufacturers of these scales promise that they measure fat mass in specific areas, muscle mass, and water retention. Many of us who have been on a set of these scales wonder how accurate they truly are.

All body fat scales use a method called bioelectrical impedance analysis (BIA). BIA is one of the quickest ways to analyze body composition. It works by sending a very low-level electrical signal through your legs or arms or both. BIA can be done through stand-on scales, a handheld device, or a combination of both. Recently, combination methods have become more popular, and many fitness centers have large scales you stand on and hold on to at the same time. By measuring the rate at which the electrical signal travels through various body tissues (fat and muscle), a BIA device can estimate body fat percentage, among other things. The downside to BIA is that it can easily be affected by your level of hydration, food intake, and even skin temperature. Beware of companies promoting these devices and claiming otherwise.

More often than not, BIA devices overestimate whole-body muscle mass and skeletal mass when compared to other gold-standard methods of measurement (Lee et al. 2018). And this overestimation would be reflected in your measurement of overall body fat percentage. For this reason, they are consistently inaccurate compared to gold-standard methods (Wang et al. 2016). Although the numbers you see when you step on these machines might not reflect your true body fat percentage, the readings will be consistent when you measure frequently. As inaccurate as they might be (up to a few percentage points of your true measurements), they will be just as inaccurate the next time you measure yourself, so you will be able to track your progress. Use them to track changes, but take the actual numbers with a grain of salt. You can increase the accuracy of these readings by taking them at the same time each day and with the same levels of hydration and food intake.

SKINFOLD CALIPERS

Some fitness and supplement companies hand out plastic body fat calipers like a toy inside a chocolate egg. More experienced trainers and professional facilities might even have giant metal ones; these often cost quite a bit more than your plastic ones and need recalibrating frequently. As far as useful and practical methods of body fat assessment go, measuring skinfolds produces some of the most accurate readings. That is, if the measurements are taken by an experienced professional and not your best friend (or you awkwardly trying to pinch your own body fat), they can be almost as accurate as a DEXA scan. The method and sites that you pinch may look simple enough, but having someone who knows what they are doing will produce far more accurate results, giving a good indication of your overall muscle and fat mass.

It is not within the scope of this book to cover the exact protocol for assessing body fat through skinfolds. But, in brief, the tester measures the thickness of your subcutaneous fat by carefully pinching skin and fat in certain areas on your body. The specific sites vary depending on the procedure and calculations used, but usually three to seven skinfold sites are chosen. The readings from these sites are put into an equation, which can be found on many websites and even mobile apps, to calculate body fat percentages. Inputting the thickness of these skinfold measurements alongside other data (typically weight and age) will produce a calculation of your body fat percentage, lean mass, and fat mass. You may also want to keep track of the skinfold thickness obtained from individual areas, such as those around your abdominals.

As a practical and accessible method of body fat assessment, this technique can be relatively accurate. However, the accuracy is highly dependent on the person taking the measurements as well as the skinfold sites and equations used (España Romero et al. 2009). If you are using skinfold calipers, measuring may be more of a monthly than a weekly occurrence. This is because weekly changes would be so small and hard to accurately measure. Use an experienced and suitably qualified professional who has accurate calipers, otherwise the readings will be inconsistent and useless.

GIRTH MEASUREMENTS

Taking girth measurements is a common practice among fitness professionals. Most of us also have experience measuring ourselves for clothes or even the size of our biceps after an arm day pump! Measuring six-pack progress with a tape measure isn't the best idea, though. However, it is a highly useful and practical way to measure changes to your overall body shape. Along with a six-pack, it is likely you want that V-taper look of a wider upper body and narrow waist. Knowing certain body measurements will give you a picture over time of what's growing and what's shrinking.

If you use this technique, do not think that building your abs will give you a bigger waist measurement. Even the highest level of physique competitors typically have waists smaller than 32 inches (81 cm)! You can measure your biceps, chest, and even glutes if you want to see how your shape is changing over time. Just don't rely on these measurements for weekly progress updates. Doing so and expecting large changes in body measurements will only cause you to believe you aren't making progress. Plus, if you don't know what measurements you're aiming for in the first place, then you won't know whether you're achieving them.

PROGRESS PHOTOS

Taking a "before" photo does not have to mean sharing a half-naked picture of yourself with friends on social media. It can mean taking pictures of yourself from different angles and storing them for comparison against future pictures. Doing this will allow you to compare progress as your body changes. If you have a coach or trainer, this can be part of the weekly or monthly check-in process. Comparing photos side by side gives great visual feedback.

Comparing pictures of what you look like today with those taken a month ago and seeing the changes can be all the motivation you need to keep going. It can be the validation you need to know that what you've been doing has been worth the effort. Or it can be an indicator that something needs to change. In both circumstances, looking at yourself in the mirror every day won't allow you to see the big changes because the daily differences are so small. Checking in with yourself or a professional once a month, or even weekly, is one of the best and easiest methods for tracking your progress. You won't know your true body fat percentage, but you will get a great indicator of how good your abs look after a few months of the workouts from this book.

Take the pictures with the same device, in the same lighting, and at the same angles. Take the photos at the same time of day and, ideally, on the same day each week. In a nutshell, just keep everything the same! Take a progress picture from the front, from the side, and from behind (see figure 5.1). Taking them both relaxed *and* flexed is useful too. Or ensure that you're flexing the same amount every time. Keep the pictures on your camera phone, email them to yourself, send them to your coach, or even send them to a partner or friend to make sure you're taking photos consistently. Taking progress photos is the best thing you can do to track your six-pack progress.

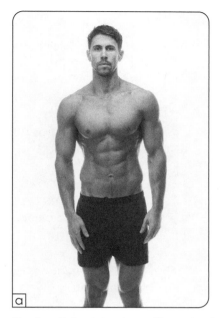
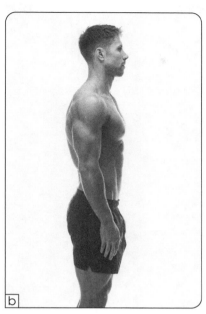
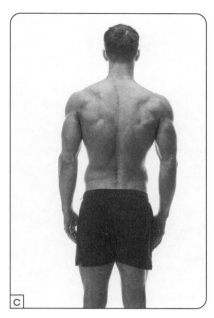

Figure 5.1   Ideal positions for tracking progress using photos. *(a)* Front to the camera and arms relaxed, *(b)* side to the camera and arms relaxed, and *(c)* back to the camera and arms relaxed.

SUMMARY

Establishing appropriate body targets is one of the most important aspects of any transformation training plan. Unrealistic expectations can cause you to want to quit early, even if the path you're on would have eventually gotten you the results you were aiming for. Everyone has the potential to achieve visible six-pack abs. Even if you perceive age or genetics to be an obstacle, you can still choose to gain better abs tomorrow than you have today. Tracking those changes helps that happen.

Overall, it's up to you to choose how to measure changes in your physique over time. This will depend on your access to equipment, access to professionals, and personal preference. It's important you understand that each method has its limitations. Still, using any of the methods in this chapter will greatly increase your chances of obtaining your ideal physique and six-pack abs.

The Exercises

Part II of this book takes you through the exercises you need to know in order to obtain aesthetic abs and an unbreakable core. Starting with chapter 6, you'll learn how to select the best exercises to give you unparalleled results while keeping you injury free. You'll understand what correct exercise technique really is, how your exercise selection is dictated by your goals (hint: narrow down!), and how to progress exercises based on your level.

Chapter 7 takes a dive into spinal flexion, how to most effectively use spinal flexion movements, and the best flexion exercises to work your abs. Every exercise in part II includes the rationale for why it works and a designated level according to its difficulty. This helps you better understand why you may or not use it within your own programming or why it might fit into one of the programs outlined in part III.

Next, in chapter 8 you'll find some of the most effective exercises and techniques you can use to target your lower abs. For many people, the lower abdominal area can be a real trouble spot. You may not be able to isolate this area, but specific exercises have been shown to preferentially recruit the lower fibers of the rectus abdominis (see chapter 3). If you're in pursuit of the fabled eight-pack, then you'll learn how to specifically target the lower portion of your abs.

The inclusion of lateral flexion and rotational movements is necessary for developing impressive obliques. In chapter 9, you'll learn some of the most effective ways to target this area. From cables to bands to landmine training, you'll find every exercise you need to chisel your obliques and build unstoppable rotational strength and power.

In chapter 3, you learned the key differences between core and ab training. In chapter 10, you'll find the most popular and useful exercises for attaining a solid core. These "anti" exercises will be a useful addition to your training for aesthetics by helping you build abs that not only look good but also perform well. There's no use in being *all show* without having *the go*! These exercises are essential for stabilizing your spine and building an unbreakable core. Chapter 10 will show you what works and how to combine core and ab training for the best results.

Finally, in chapter 11, you'll learn the six exercises you need to complement your ab training. These exercises contribute to spinal health and injury prevention from a biomechanics perspective and can work alongside your ab and core exercises to build an impressive overall physique. You'll find a specific focus on glute, lumbar, and adductor exercises. Some of these exercises are popular, while others are commonly neglected, which makes certain muscles an area of weakness for many people. Refer to this section anytime you need exercise inspiration or to keep your training fresh or just as a reminder that you do have other muscles besides the ones that look good in the mirror.

Selecting the Best Exercises

It is common to be bombarded daily with information telling you what the best exercises are for X or Y body part. What most of that information won't tell you is that the best exercises are specific to you, your body type, and your training history. What might be the best exercise for one person could be the worst for another. This chapter will help you narrow your goals and teach you how to select the exercises that are best for you. In doing so, you will achieve better and faster results and even eliminate injuries and pain.

NARROWING YOUR GOALS

In chapters 2 and 3, we discussed abdominal anatomy and how *function* dictates exercise selection. We know that combining spinal flexion, posterior pelvic tilt, rotation, lateral flexion, and the "anti" exercises is important if you want to build a solid core and six-pack abs. This knowledge can be overwhelming when it's time to select exercises, though. And while structuring your training to cover all of these functions is important in the long run, when it comes to developing chiseled abs, it's important that exercises be prioritized. Quite simply, you want to spend the most time on exercises that will reap the fastest results.

When selecting the best exercises, it's important to remind yourself of your priorities right now. The more you can narrow your goals, the better your final list of exercises will be. For example, developing core strength and using "anti" exercises to help increase spinal stability are important. And the exercises that accomplish this tend to be more interesting than other exercises. Despite wanting to include them in your list of go-to exercises, right now your goals are primarily based on appearance. Therefore, right now, a larger ratio of your exercises should be focused on the goal of looking good in the mirror. As superficial as that might sound, the more you train for this, the closer you'll get to your ideal body. Then, once you've achieved your aesthetic goals, your priorities might change to include more injury-prevention and performance-based exercises.

The ratio of exercises changes, and which exercises are best changes as well. The best exercises are relative, and an exercise is only the best choice if it will get you from where you are right now to where you want to be. You will learn how to narrow your exercise choices to those that are best for *you*. You'll also learn which exercises to delete from your training toolbox forever, and how by doing so you'll save yourself a lot of time and wasted energy in the process.

TRAINING VERSUS WORKING OUT

By selecting the best exercises, you'll save time, move better, experience less unwanted pain, and get closer to achieving your ultimate goal of impressive six-pack abs. This is why it's important you learn how to select the best exercises for you, so you can direct your efforts in the right direction within your training.

One of the biggest misconceptions about exercise is that effort equates to results. There's nothing more admirable than watching someone put their blood, sweat, and tears into a workout and getting after it. Watching another person with that amount of drive uplifts the energy in the entire room, causing you to work a bit harder, too. But working out hard doesn't necessarily mean working out smart or that you're following a specific and structured training plan.

To work out can simply imply throwing a bunch of exercises together for the purpose of getting tired and sweaty—something you can put your efforts into and feel great about at the end but won't necessarily guarantee progress. Anyone can put together a single workout that will make then tired at the end, but the programs in this book put you through a purposeful training *experience*.

Training implies that you're on a path toward something bigger than what happens in a single workout or during a set of a randomly assigned exercises. Training is a specific process of progression. It's meaningful and purposeful training that produces measurable or visual results. One of the first steps toward building structure within your training is understanding how to progress and regress exercises and how to select the best exercises for you.

WHY IS TECHNIQUE IMPORTANT?

Exercise technique can be broken into two key areas. For each of the exercises covered in part II, exercise *setup* and exercise *performance* are described in detail. This will help you optimize the technique to get the best results from each exercise.

Exercise Setup

Exercise setup describes the correct position of your body and of the equipment you'll use before starting the exercise. The position of the equipment is important, as is aligning your body and the weights in the safest and most effective way possible. A setup that is even a little off can result in slight awkwardness, complete joint misalignment, or even injury. If an exercise is more awkward than it should be, you'll enjoy it less and won't be as likely to do it consistently. Resistance that is misaligned with your joints and other structures can result in wear and tear, potential damage, and an inefficient position in which your muscles can't activate to their full capacity. We can use the very simple example of a door hinge and compare it to that of the hinge of your elbow joint. If you repeatedly try to pull a door in a direction it isn't designed to travel in, over time, even small amounts of this force would result in a poorly functioning hinge. Applying larger misaligned forces would result in a bent hinge or even rip the door completely off the hinge. In the human body, this can be compared to misaligned triceps exercises resulting in flareups or epicondylitis (tennis or golfer's elbow). The same holds true for every other joint, including those within your spine. Taking your time to set up for each exercise correctly will put you in better alignment to achieve results and longevity.

Exercise Performance

Also termed *exercise execution*, exercise performance describes the motion that's happening when the actual movement is taking place after correct setup has been established. For example, once you've set yourself in position on the floor to do an abdominal crunch, the performance of the exercise is when you begin to crunch upward. Compare this to the performance on a theater stage, for example. Everything on stage might be in the right position to set you up for success, but the acting and moving parts are what make that show. Utmost attention and focus on execution are paramount to your success. Each movement (repetition) that takes place should begin and finish with focus and intent toward achieving a very specific goal. As each repetition progresses, fatigue sets in and this becomes harder to maintain. The initial setup checkpoints begin to migrate, technique gets sloppy, and your focus shifts from feeling the muscle work as it should to just getting it done. For more performance-based goals, this external focus can be useful, but for aesthetic goals, the focus should be more internal and with great awareness of the muscles themselves. You will get faster results by working hard to maintain proper body positioning and performance while feeling the exercise where you should. It will also help you remain injury free.

EXERCISE PROGRESSION AND REGRESSION

If an exercise does not feel right to you, then you need to know how to adapt it or whether an alternative exercise might work better. Even when you know your technique is correct, you may still experience pain or discomfort, or the exercise just might be too difficult or heavy for you. Understanding the simple laws of exercise progression (making it harder) and regression (making it easier) will allow you to structure the most effective training approach, not just for your abdominals but for the rest of your body as well. Understanding how to progress or regress an exercise will also give you a deeper understanding of the programs in part III. You'll be able to customize these programs according to your body structure, training background, and injury history. Knowing how to progress and regress exercises will also enhance your training experience and confidence to keep your motivation at an all-time high. Five key variables influence exercise progression and regression.

Resistance (Intensity)

To make an exercise more difficult, you can apply more resistance. To make an exercise easier, you can use less resistance. Resistance change can come in many formats from changing the weight of a dumbbell or the weight on a cable stack to more complex methods such as altering your body position and other leverage factors. It might sound obvious, but making small changes in resistance can have a huge impact on how an exercise feels and the benefits you receive from it. If the resistance is too high, then your attention might shift away from technique and feeling it where you should, to an externally driven goal like how much weight you're lifting or the number of reps you're able to achieve with poor form. Using a resistance that is too low will not elicit a strong enough signal for your muscles to adapt to and get stronger from. Progressing resistance is important, but for the goal of aesthetics it should not be at the expense of losing muscular tension or performing reps without focus. Finding the right balance in the resistance you use is important.

Range of Motion

Each exercise you do has a maximum available range of motion. We could go one step further by stating that each exercise has a maximum available *pain-free* range of motion. That is, just because you see an exercise done in a certain way and with a certain range of motion, it does not mean that you should also be fitting yourself into that same mold—especially if despite having the range of motion available, the position causes pain or discomfort. A barbell deadlift is a good example. You might think you need to deadlift from the floor because it's what's accepted as being the correct full range of motion. But, if your natural body structure isn't built for it or you have a history of back pain, deadlifting directly off the floor could do you more harm than good. More back or hip pain might cause you to think that your core is weak, when in reality all you needed to do was accept that deadlifting from the floor wasn't a good fit to start off with. Next time, you might try deadlifting one or two inches (2-5 cm) off the floor to see whether it makes a difference (reduced range of motion), and then throw some extra core work on top for good measure. Increasing or decreasing range of motion can make exercises harder or easier as well as prevent pain. There are also strength and aesthetic benefits from spending more time in certain ranges of motion, so don't always consider less range of motion to be easier and therefore less effective. When viewing the exercises in part II, these are shown using a full range of motion, but don't be afraid to reduce your range of motion if you need to for any reason.

Stability

A typical path of progression often spoken about is from stable to unstable exercises. However, stating that something unstable is a progression of a more stable version and therefore a goal to aim for is inaccurate. While increasing instability does make many exercises more difficult, the question is whether the progression is making the exercise harder in the right way and according to your goals. In chapter 2, we touched on the use of unstable exercises and how adding instability can reduce an exercise's ability to target a muscle. With increased stability, you can achieve higher targeted-muscle output. So, although adding instability could be seen as a way to add progression to an exercise, you need to first consider whether that is the path of progression you should take. In the context of physique enhancement and aesthetics, progressing from a stable to unstable environment is rarely useful.

Speed

Advancing slower repetitions to faster ones isn't a progression pathway employed in this book. Faster and more explosive repetitions are usually reserved for performance-based training and enhanced athleticism. For your abdominals to receive the right signals to get stronger and build new muscle tissue, they need to be subjected to high levels of mechanical tension. This requires placing high force through the muscle tissues for longer durations than those used in power-based exercises. When repetition speed is high, it is usually at the expense of placing higher force through these tissues for periods long enough to elicit the adaptation you want. Higher repetition speeds can also take you out of optimal alignment, keeping you from getting the most from each repetition and potentially increasing the likelihood of excessive wear and tear or injury. The higher the repetition speed, the better your muscles have to be at absorbing the resistances you use as well. While increasing repetition speed can be seen as a progression, it is best reserved for when your goal shifts to performance after achieving your primary goal of aesthetics. If you are new to an exercise, it makes sense to be more cautious with repetition speed as you're learning the exercise. Even once you're past the learning stage, you should use a repetition speed that still allows you to feel the exercise working the target area. Any exercise in part II that requires you to use a specific repetition speed will be noted within the technical points of each exercise.

Body Position

Changing body position is a method of progression that largely works through the manipulation of the lever arm length. Changing leverage factors can change how much resistance you receive as a percentage of your body weight. A simple example is to use a basic front plank performed on your knees versus on your toes. Because the lever arm is longer when you're on your toes, it is a more difficult position to hold and requires your muscles to work harder. In this case, you would select the plank variation that best fits your current level of strength. Another example is performing a basic crunch. Having your arms straight and overhead is harder than having your arms by your sides. This again is an example of a simple change in lever length that adjusts the difficulty of the exercise based on changing the arm position alone. Here, the weight of your arms taken farther overhead increases the difficulty of the crunch. Exercise biomechanics can be a complex topic, but having a few go-to tricks to make an exercise easier or harder by changing your body position can serve you well. Changing body position to manipulate leverage factors is a continuing theme in part III. It's also worth noting that a change in placement of an external weight, for example a dumbbell or kettlebell, can change the difficulty of an exercise. Progression or regression of exercises using this technique will be covered as they become applicable in part III.

EXERCISE MODIFICATION

Exercise modification is a term usually used interchangeably with *exercise progression* and *regression*. However, they are different. Exercise progression and regression make an exercise program easier or harder according to a set pathway of progression (i.e., this exercise must be done before progressing to that one). However, rather than following an established order, each person's path is specific to their goals and other individual factors. Progression is never clear at the start of a training plan, even to an experienced coach or trainer. This is why having the tools to know when and how to progress and regress exercises is important as you go along.

Exercise modification is "staying in the same place" as far as exercise progression goes (i.e., this could be using the same exercise), but modifying it to improve the setup or execution experience. Knowing how to do this can turn an exercise that's uncomfortable or painful into one that's well aligned and enables you to maximally load the muscle. As an example, a modification to a crunch is using an abdominal mat under your lumbar spine to enhance the feedback and put you in a different position. This isn't a new exercise, but instead it uses a slight tweak to the original so that the crunch works better for you. Using a pad under your back knee when you're kneeling with one knee on the floor (referred to as a half-kneeling position) is another example. This might put your pelvis in a more level and stable position. You'll find specific examples of this in the half-kneeling exercises featured in chapter 10.

Exercise modification is looking at body position and alignment to see whether it can be improved. While it's true that an experienced trainer has a coaching eye and can spot when this needs to be done, you have the ability to do it, too. All it requires is awareness of your own body position and alignment when setting up and performing an exercise. If an exercise doesn't feel comfortable, it might be that the exercise isn't suited to you, or it might just be that the exercise requires a little modification. Don't be afraid to use the tools available in your surroundings to modify the exercises in part II. That is, if something helps you get in a better position, feel an exercise more, or avoid pain, anything is worth a try. It can be as simple as a slight change in body or resistance angle, propping up a limb with a foam pad, or trying a different piece of exercise equipment. When it comes to exercise modification, don't be afraid to break the rules—especially if it gets you better results while remaining injury free.

EXPLAINING EXERCISE LEVELS

Each exercise in part II is assigned a level. As you might already gather from your understanding of exercise progression, levels of exercise is a more complex topic than some would have you believe. This is because determining levels is more of an art than an exact science. One school of thought is that exercise levels are assigned based on your resistance training experience. Someone might suggest that you are a beginner, intermediate, or advanced lifter based on how long you've been training. The exact number of years it takes to become an experienced lifter varies, but it tends to fall between 2 and 10 years of consistent training. There are many problems with assigning exercises and suggesting certain repetition ranges and volumes based on this assumption, but the biggest comes from the fact that your level is more exercise specific than person specific. That is, you could have accumulated vast experience and mastery of one exercise but be a complete beginner on another.

Maybe you practice powerlifting, and you're highly experienced at the barbell back squat. You've spent years under that bar for hours each week trying to perfect your technique. But unless you've spent an equal amount of time doing Bulgarian split squats, you will not be as proficient at them. You may be able to transfer some strength and skill to them, but your level will not be the same. This is true no matter whether we are talking about something as complex as an Olympic lift or as simple as a biceps curl. Levels of exercises are relative to how much experience you have doing them and how suited your body is to performing them.

To some people, a basic abdominal crunch is a foundational exercise. That's because it has relatively low complexity and high stability, it's an isolated exercise, and you're typically using your own body weight. But it actually takes a lot of body awareness to be able to master a basic crunch in a way that it will effectively work your abdominals. A kettlebell windmill has a higher level of complexity and requires you hold a weight overhead, which can be more dangerous for some people. But experience tells you that if a kettlebell windmill were shown to someone with a dance background, they'd hit all the positional requirements on their first attempt. This could be despite never having picked up a kettlebell before. The level of an exercise is relative to the person doing it and not necessarily based on their experience or years of training.

In part II, you'll see each exercise assigned with a perceived level of difficulty. This level of difficulty is based on the level of complexity of the exercise and typically the time it takes to teach the exercise. Exercises with low complexity might be presented in picture format and can be mimicked almost immediately. These exercises might be classified as foundational or intermediate, but this does not mean that you should skip the performance steps just because you consider yourself more advanced. Exercises assigned to each category are done to give you a starting guide for what to expect from each exercise. If you're new to this, then you will most likely benefit from spending your time on foundational exercises and beginner programs. If you have experience, you might still want to start at the foundational or intermediate levels, but advance to more challenging exercises and programs more quickly. In both examples, the aim is to master your setup and execution before doing the same with higher-level exercises.

For physique development and the goal of attaining impressive abdominals, the following definitions and classifications are used in part III:

• *Foundational:* These exercises have low complexity and require very little teaching time. These exercises involve a single joint action and therefore have a single focus. For example, focusing on spinal flexion during a basic crunch is classified as a foundational movement and exercise.

• *Intermediate:* These exercises are more complex and require more teaching time than a foundational exercise, but they have less complexity than an advanced exercise. These exercises still involve very few joint actions, but they require a little more thought during performance.

• *Advanced:* These exercises are typically multijoint and require greater levels of strength to perform. With higher complexity and more thought required, the focus moves away from feeling the muscles working and toward an external goal like completing the movement or achieving a certain number of repetitions. Advanced exercises should be used only if an internal focus can be maintained.

• *Hardcore:* These exercises require the greatest levels of strength and have the highest levels of complexity. These exercises challenge you and make you work hard. Do not mistake the ability to do these as your final goal. Instead, see them as a way to keep your training interesting, or when you *do* have the capacity, to take it up a level.

Captain Crunch: Targeting Your Spine

As mentioned in chapter 2, little scientific evidence shows that repeated spinal flexion poses risk to your back health. This is especially true for exercises that don't involve spinal flexion and compression at the same time. In previous chapters, we presented arguments for and against the use of spinal flexion exercises such as crunches. It is your choice whether or not to use the exercises presented in this chapter. However, remember that when done correctly, spinal flexion exercises can form part of a complete approach to training strong and chiseled abs. Most exercises are very low risk and including them in your routine can be greatly rewarding.

To get six-pack abs, it's essential you learn how to isolate and target your rectus abdominis in the most effective way possible. Creating large amounts of mechanical tension by placing load across those muscle tissues is key.

Trying to develop your six-pack without spinal flexion exercises is like trying to build bigger biceps without performing biceps curls. Sure, you can hit your biceps with multijoint exercises such as chin-ups, but you will not create enough targeted load across your biceps to build them most efficiently. This is especially true if you have a stubborn muscle that needs extra attention. The rules for bigger biceps are the same for etching out six-pack abs.

While multijoint and core exercises are important, learning how to isolate your rectus abdominis with flexion-based exercises are just as important.

Crunches and similar exercises should be part of an intelligent approach to your abs training. You need to know the best exercises and how to execute them correctly in order to get the most from them. Gone are the days of performing hundreds of crunches. You deserve better.

A NOTE ON BREATHING

Your breath is a powerful tool. From changing your nervous system state to feeling either more energized, or in a state of relaxation, to helping get the most out of each repetition, your breath is a great influencer. As a general rule your inhalation (inward breath) should be performed during the "easiest" portion of the exercise. This is typically the eccentric or downward phase. Your outward breath should be on the "effort," which is typically the concentric or lifting phase.

Nasal breathing should be encouraged as much as possible (in through the nose and out through the nose), although breathing in through the nose and out through the mouth is also acceptable and easier for most. To feel the difference a breath makes, try performing a basic abdominal crunch while exhaling fully at the top as you simultaneously contract your abdominals as hard as possible. Then, try doing the same thing while using only shallow breaths, or holding your breath entirely. The contraction in the former will be far greater while making for a more efficient workout overall. Some of the exercises in this chapter mention the use of breath, just in case you need the reminder.

1
BASIC ABDOMINAL CRUNCH

Level: Foundational

There is nothing basic about performing basic abdominal crunches—providing you're doing them right, that is. Use basic crunch variations to isolate your abs effectively and strike your target efficiently. Until you know how to perform a basic crunch in the most effective way, you won't get the most from other integrated exercises.

You must have a laser focus on what you're trying to achieve from each repetition. This requires you to develop an internal focus. This means thinking about the isolated action you're performing, the muscle you're targeting, and creating maximal tension in that area. Set up correctly, stabilize, pull your ribs toward your pelvis, and contract your abs hard—as hard as you can. Once you can create tension on every rep, you can introduce a little weight.

Setup

- Lie on a mat for comfort with your knees bent, head down, and hands behind your ears (optional).
- As an option, you can place a small rolled-up towel under your lower back for support.

Performance

1. Imagine a tennis ball between your chin and chest the entire time, maintaining a neutral neck.
2. Begin the crunch by pulling your rib cage down toward your pelvis as you lift your shoulders off the floor.
3. Close the space between your ribs and pelvis by also pulling your pelvis upward a little at the same time (a posterior tilt of your pelvis).

4. Rise as high as you can until you can no longer flex your spine. If you flex your hips to come up higher, you've come up too far.

5. Maintaining abdominal tension throughout each repetition, lower yourself fully to the floor, this time opening the space between your ribs and pelvis to take your abdominals through as great a stretch as possible.

6. As you rise, attempt to exhale fully while taking a breath in on the way back down.

Tips for Success

- Hand position during basic body-weight crunches matters more than you think.
- Because of a longer lever arm length, performing crunches with your hands by your sides is easier than with them on your chest.
- Putting your hands on your head or behind your ears is even more difficult, while straightening your arms and holding them higher over your head is the hardest.
- Use this information to make your crunches easier or harder by manipulating your body leverages.
- You can also perform a drop set: Start the set with your hands highest, and then as you fatigue bring them closer to your sides to finish.

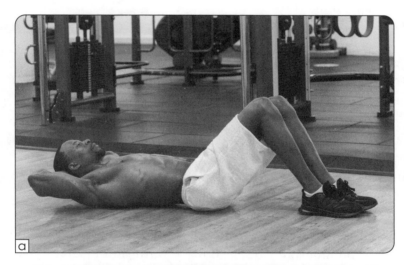

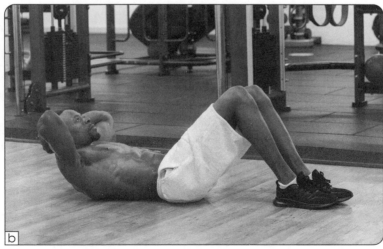

2
STABILITY BALL CRUNCH

Level: Intermediate

These crunches add a stability ball to your basic crunch technique. A stability ball is sometimes seen as unstable-surface training, but its use here is less about that and more about the shape of the ball itself. While the unstable nature of the stability ball might help to activate other stabilizer muscles around your hips and spine, it's the curvature of the ball that benefits your six-pack training the most. The curve of the stability ball should sit in the natural curve of your lower back, creating the perfect environment to target your rectus abdominis through a greater range of motion.

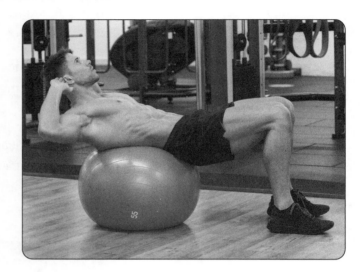

Setup

- Select the correct size stability ball according to manufacturer instructions.
- Lie on the stability ball with the curve of your lower back resting on the highest point of the ball. Roll the ball a few inches up or down to find the point where you're most balanced.
- Your knees should be about hip-width apart and bent 90 degrees, and your feet are firmly planted on the floor.
- Place your hands behind your ears or on your chest.

Performance

1. Imagine a tennis ball between your chin and chest the entire time, maintaining a neutral neck.
2. Begin the crunch by pulling your rib cage down toward your pelvis as you lift your shoulders.
3. Close the space between your ribs and pelvis by also pulling your pelvis upward a little at the same time (a posterior tilt of your pelvis). Your lower back should be pressed into the ball the entire time.
4. Contract your abdominals as hard as you can as you lift, exhaling fully as you approach the top.
5. Do not flex your hips at the top. Full concentric range of motion is when you can no longer flex your spine.
6. Lower fully using the curvature of the stability ball to guide you, getting as much extension over the ball as possible. This allows a full and intense stretch of your abdominals.
7. Maintain abdominal tension from start to finish.

Tips for Success

- For some people, the unstable nature of using a stability ball can hinder the goal of creating targeted muscle tension.
- Generally, creating a more stable environment will produce better results for muscle development.
- In place of a stability ball, ask a partner to hold and stabilize you from your knees, or set up so your knees are pressed into a wall to lock you in.

3
CABLE STABILITY BALL CRUNCH

Level: Advanced

Cable stability ball crunches are an effective way to add load to standard stability ball crunches. Using a cable creates a more constant resistance. Because of the angle of the cable, a longer lever length is hardest at the top of the crunch where your rectus abdominis is in a fully shortened position. This makes it a very effective six-pack builder.

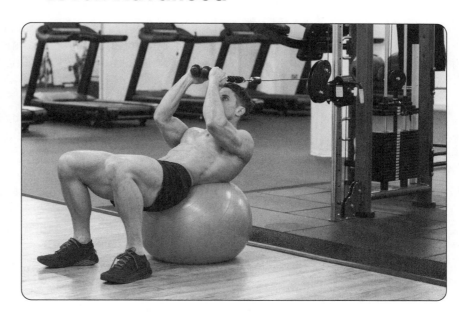

Setup

- Select the correct size stability ball according to manufacturer instructions.
- Set the cable height a little higher than the height of your shoulders when lying on the ball. Ideally, the angle between your torso and the cable at the top of the crunch is approximately 90 degrees. Achieving this may take some trial and error.
- Use a dual-rope attachment on your cable system.
- Holding the rope attachment, lie on the stability ball with the highest point of the ball resting in the curve of your lower back. Roll the ball a few inches up or down to find the point where you're most balanced.
- Position yourself and the ball far enough away from the cable stack to allow a full range of motion in the crunch when using the cables.
- Hold the dual-rope attachment to your shoulders, or if it's more comfortable, you can also keep them close together and slightly overhead.

Performance

1. Keeping the rope firmly in position, begin to crunch upward.
2. Pull your ribs down toward your pelvis, allowing the cable resistance to load you as you do so.
3. Use only a small amount of cable resistance to start. You don't want excessive load to distract you from an internal focus; maximal abdominal tension should be felt throughout the exercise.
4. Exhale fully as you reach the top.
5. Lower to the start, using the stability ball to allow a full range of motion at the bottom.

Tips for Success

If you don't have access to a cable system, a resistance band is just as effective when it is set to the same height as shown with the cables.

4

HAMSTRING-ACTIVATED SIT-UP

Level: Advanced

Activating your hamstrings can make your abs work harder by causing a reciprocal inhibition of your hip flexors. Stopping your hip flexors from working in your sit-ups and even in crunches forces your rectus abdominis and external obliques to do the majority of the lifting.

Setup

Set up to perform a regular crunch or sit-up by firmly pressing your heels against an immovable weightlifting platform, the edge of a thick mat, or even the hands of a partner.

Performance

1. Drive your heels into the object to engage your hamstrings; keep them engaged throughout the set.
2. Begin by lifting your shoulders off the floor and flexing your spine to maximally contract your abdominals. This will be harder than you first thought.
3. Reach the end of the crunch and continue to flex your hips further into a full sit-up.
4. Imagine a tennis ball between your chin and chest the entire time, maintaining a neutral neck.
5. Once you reach the top, lower yourself under control, taking two to four seconds to come all the way down.

Tips for Success

The concept of activating your hamstrings to increase abdominal activation was popularized by Vladimir Janda, a Czech neurologist, physical therapist, and teacher. Similar versions of these are often called Janda sit-ups.

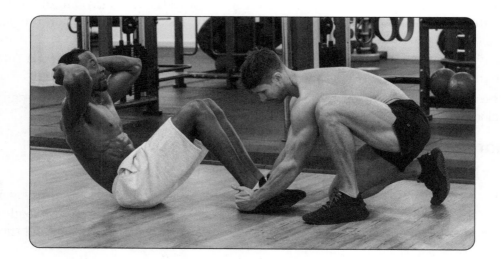

5
HAMSTRING-ACTIVATED STABILITY BALL CRUNCH

Level: Advanced

The hamstring-activated stability ball crunch combines the benefits of using a stability ball with the act of engaging your hamstrings while performing a crunch. While the stability ball increases the range of motion, activating your hamstrings will help deactivate your hip flexors somewhat, causing your abdominals to work a bit harder.

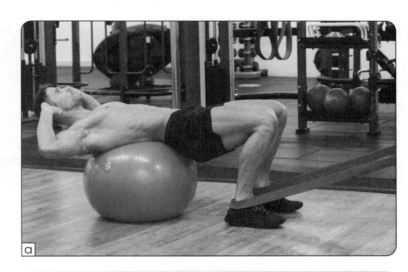

Setup

- Press your heels into a resistance band or the edge of a weightlifting platform or thick rubber mat.
- Select the correct size stability ball according to manufacturer instructions.
- Lie on the stability ball as if to perform a basic stability ball crunch.

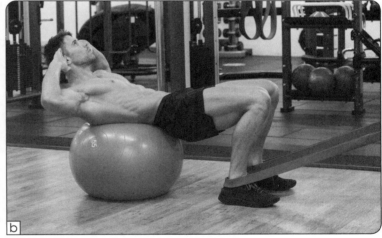

Performance

1. Drive your heels into the immovable object to engage your hamstrings, and maintain hamstring tension throughout the set.

2. Simultaneously pull your ribs toward your hips to maximally contract your abdominals. Do this with your hands placed over your abdominals to help increase awareness.

3. Reach the top of the crunch, and then lower under control. Be sure to get full extension of your abdominals over the stability ball.

Tips for Success

- The main difference between a crunch and a sit-up is the additional flexion of your hips that is needed to reach the top of a full sit-up.
- One might argue that because your abdominals don't act to flex your hips, overall a crunch is superior to a sit-up for abdominal development.

6
LYING BANDED CRUNCH

Level: Intermediate

Much like using a cable during a crunch, a resistance band can effectively load your crunches. If you're short on equipment or space, all you need is a floor and resistance band to take your basic crunch to the next level.

Setup

- Use a floor mat for comfort (optional).
- Loop a resistance band around a sturdy object.
- Lie with your knees bent, head on the mat, and hands clenching the band.
- The resistance band should be parallel to your head and held either close to your shoulders or just over the top of your forehead.
- Keep resistance in the band, even at the bottom of your crunch.

Performance

1. Begin the crunch by pulling your rib cage toward your pelvis as you lift your shoulders off the floor.
2. Close the space between your ribs and pelvis by also pulling your pelvis upward a little at the same time (a posterior tilt of your pelvis).
3. As you rise, the resistance from the band will increase.
4. Rise as high as you can until you can no longer flex your spine.
5. Maintain maximal abdominal tension as you lower yourself fully.
6. Do not let the band slacken at the bottom.

Tips for Success

- Sometimes a single resistance band is all you need in your travel bag for a good ab workout.
- Vary the band's resistance by starting with more or less stretch or holding it in different positions.

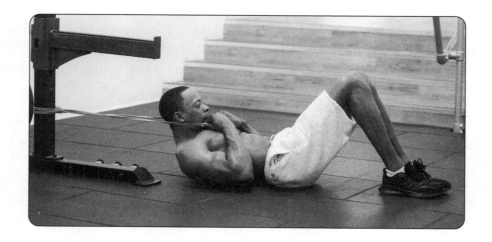

7
LYING BANDED ELBOWS TO KNEES

Level: Intermediate

This exercise is a form of double crunch. A double crunch involves doing a crunch while holding your feet off the floor, which places your pelvis in a more posterior tilt, allowing the abdominals to contract harder at the top. Use a resistance band for next-level difficulty.

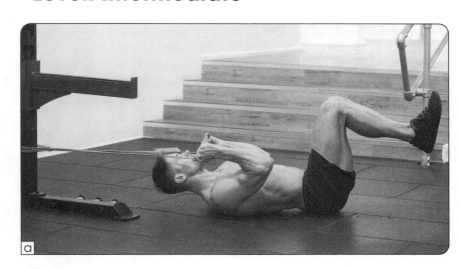

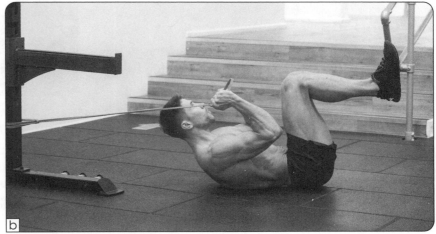

Setup

- Loop a resistance band around a sturdy object.
- Lie on the floor with the resistance band above your head.
- Keep your knees bent to about 90 degrees and lift your feet off the floor.
- Imagine pushing your lower back into the floor and scooping your pelvis up toward your hips (posterior pelvic tilt).

Performance

1. Keeping the band overhead or close to your shoulders, begin your crunch.
2. Pull your ribs down toward your pelvis, keeping your abs as tense as possible.
3. As you rise, the band resistance will increase.
4. Attempt to touch your elbows to your knees by allowing your knees to tuck closer in as you reach the top of the crunch.
5. Lower while keeping your feet off the floor.

Tips for Success

- Lying elbows to knees can be done with a cable pulley.
- Use a dual-rope attachment for the most comfort when holding.

8
STANDING HEAVY-BAND CRUNCH

Level: Foundational

Standing heavy-band crunches aren't just for your garage gym or limited-equipment workouts. Using a resistance band increases resistance as you flex farther into your crunch. Increased tension as your abdominals shorten gives useful feedback on how your abs should feel when contracting hard. For a maximum ab workout, finding ways to create tension in this fully flexed position is key.

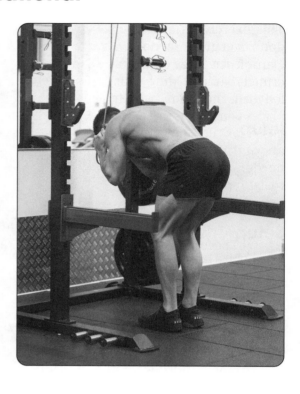

Setup

- Loop a single resistance band around something high, such as a pull-up bar or a wooden beam.
- Stand directly under the band.
- Keep your knees soft.

Performance

1. Shorten the band as needed. The higher on the band you hold and the more you stretch it, the more resistance you'll create.
2. Bend forward into a crunch, tensing your abs hard.
3. Experiment with stepping farther in or away from the band to create a different feeling during the crunches.
4. The band stretches, making the bottom of the crunch even more difficult.
5. Maintain maximal abdominal tension throughout. Don't be afraid to start with the band a little looser if it means you can feel it more.

Tips for Success

- Bands provide an easy drop set opportunity.
- Start your set with the band held shorter, and then as you fatigue, let the band slacken and keep going.
- An inch or two difference in where you hold the band can feel like a significant drop in weight.

9

KNEELING CABLE CRUNCH

Level: Foundational

Kneeling cable crunches are a commonly performed gym exercise used to develop six-pack abs. They're also commonly performed incorrectly. Decrease the weight, and focus on optimal execution.

Setup

- Use a dual-rope attachment or V-bar attachment on your cable system.
- Set the cable height so you can grab it from a kneeling position while retaining resistance in the cable. This will vary according to your height.
- Position yourself about half a body length from the cable and grab hold of it.

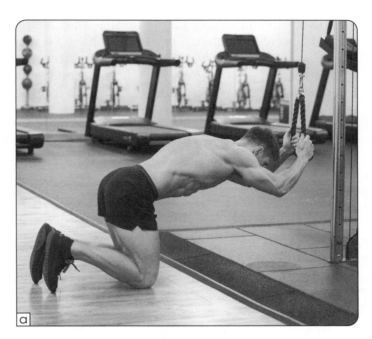

Performance

1. Hold the cable just over the top of your head and try to keep it there through the duration of the exercise. You can also hold it over your shoulders if it's more comfortable.

2. In your kneeling position, lean in toward the cable, allowing the resistance on the cable to hold you up.

3. Keep your hips stacked over your knees at all times. Your thighs must remain nearly vertical while you're flexing into your crunch. Avoid the common mistake of shifting your hips back as you do your cable crunches.

4. Pull your ribs to your pelvis, closing the space between these two points and flexing your abs hard.

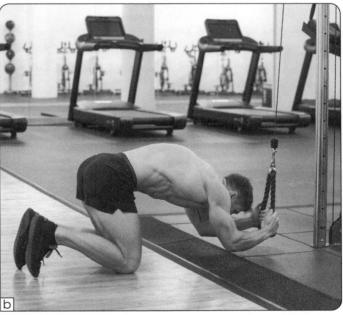

5. Come all the way out of the crunch by stretching your abdominals, but do not move your hips.

6. Exhale fully as you flex into your crunch, and inhale as you come up.

Tips for Success

Using a foam pad for your knees not only increases comfort, but it also provides a marker to aim your elbows toward as you crunch down, as well as keeping your range of motion consistent.

10
STANDING CABLE CRUNCH

Level: Intermediate

Standing cable crunches can be done either facing toward the cable stack or away from it. Each version loads you in different ways. When facing away from the cable stack you feel the exercise more in the middle of the movement; facing toward the cable you'll feel the bottom of the crunch more. Perform whichever method feels the best for you and will provide the desired results. Here's how to do them facing away from the cables to work the top of the movement.

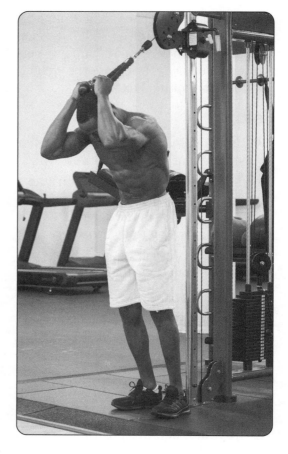

Setup

- Use a dual-rope attachment on a single cable.
- Set the cable high.
- Stand with your back to the cable column and the rope attachment over your shoulders.

Performance

1. Standing cable crunches are more like sit-ups than crunches.
2. Keeping the cable close to your shoulders, begin by contracting your abs hard and flexing your spine, almost as if you're bowing forward but with a flexed spine.
3. As you reach full spinal flexion, continue with a little flexion of your hip to finish off the movement.
4. Return to the start position, but keep your abs engaged.

Tips for Success

Because the design of cable systems varies, standing with your back to some of them can become awkward. If this is the case, use a lat pull-down machine. Simply fix a dual-rope attachment and stand with the seat between your legs and your back toward the knee rest.

11
LANDMINE CRUNCH

Level: Advanced

Your abdominals require progressive overload over time just like every other muscle in your body. This is what causes them to adapt and become stronger. Landmine crunches are a novel way to add extra load to your crunches and continue your progression.

Setup

- Position yourself on the floor with the landmine between your legs.
- Press the landmine and keep your elbows fully extended throughout.
- You may require trial and error to feel the movement and find the position that feels best for you.

Performance

1. With your elbows straight, begin to lift your shoulders off the floor, pushing the landmine upward.
2. The landmine will dictate your path of movement.
3. Keep your feet firmly pressed into the floor as you perform your crunch.
4. Pull the rib cage toward your pelvis and contract your abdominals as hard as you can.

Tips for Success

The design of a landmine unit makes it fractionally heavier at the bottom of the movement than at the top. You can use this information to apply more or less resistance in a certain portion of an exercise to either work a muscle differently or prevent a potentially awkward or painful range of motion.

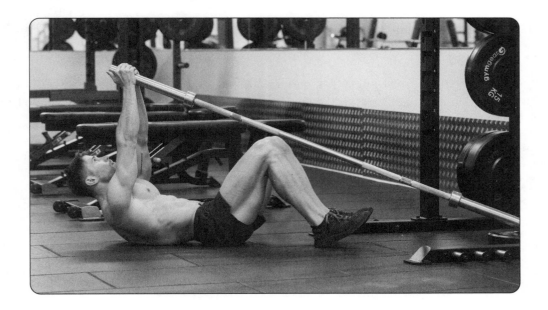

12

CRUNCH WITH A LAT PULL-DOWN MACHINE

Level: Advanced

Crunches can be effectively loaded using most lat pull-down cables. The advantage is that sitting under the knee support keeps you locked in, enabling you to focus more on working the target area.

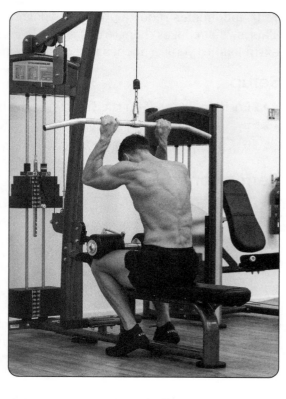

Setup

- Adjust the height of the knee support so you can lock your knees under.
- Hold the lat pull-down bar attachment with a narrow overhand grip.
- Start with a light weight on the cables until you get used to it.

Performance

1. Pull your knees into the knee support as you pull the bar down. Activate your lats as you pull to create as much tension as possible before initiating the actual crunching movement.
2. Keeping the bar overhead, crunch down, pulling your rib cage toward the floor.
3. Your elbows may touch the knee support.
4. Hold the bottom for a split second and squeeze your abs hard before coming back up.

Tips for Success

Generally speaking, the more stability you can create within an exercise the more output you can get from a targeted muscle. In other words, you can isolate it more efficiently. At the same time, this can be at the expense of stabilizer muscle activation. Pick the right tools for the job.

13
INCLINE ECCENTRIC CABLE CRUNCH

Level: Hardcore

In chapter 1 you learned that eccentric contractions are the motion of an active muscle while lengthening under load. Eccentric training is one of the best forms of exercise for building muscle. It can create large amounts of mechanical tension and tissue breakdown, both powerful triggers of muscle hypertrophy. Incline eccentric cable crunches are a good way to apply eccentric training to your abdominals. They overload the eccentric portion of the crunch by putting you in a mechanically disadvantageous position as you lower yourself (holding the cable farther overhead makes them more difficult). As you perform the upward crunch, you'll do so with more ease (because holding the cable closer to your body is easier).

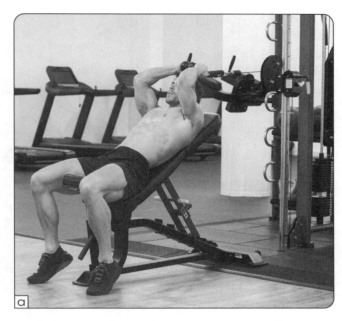

Setup

- Position a bench at an approximately 30- to 45-degree incline. Use the incline that works best for you.
- Use a dual-rope attachment on the cable set a little higher than the height of the bench backrest.
- Sit on the bench and pull the rope in close over your shoulders.

Performance

1. Keeping the rope close to your shoulders, begin to crunch, pulling your elbows down toward your hips.
2. Hold the top for a brief second, and press the rope away from your shoulders farther overhead. The larger distance the rope is from your body will make it harder for your abdominals to resist.

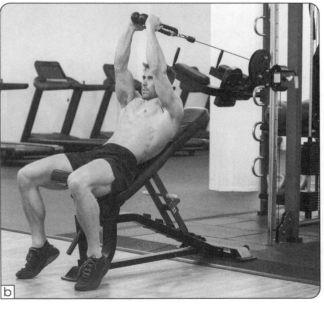

3. Fight the weight as you lower yourself with control to the start position. Take two to four seconds to get there.

Tips for Success

Your eccentric strength can be 20 to 40 percent greater than your concentric strength. This means that as your abs contract and shorten, they have less capacity to lift weight than when they are lengthening. You can capitalize on this extra strength by making an exercise harder to perform on the way down than on the way up.

14
ABDOMINAL V-UP

Level: Intermediate

Abdominal V-ups are basic but brilliant. They combine a body-weight crunch with a leg raise. You could say they're more of a complete six-pack exercise than performing crunches alone. These are suitable for all levels.

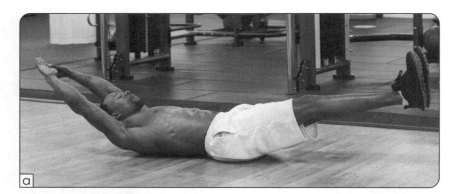

Setup

- Lie faceup on the floor. Your arms are overhead, knees straight, and feet together.

- To maintain tension throughout, start and finish each repetition with your arms and feet hovering just off the floor.

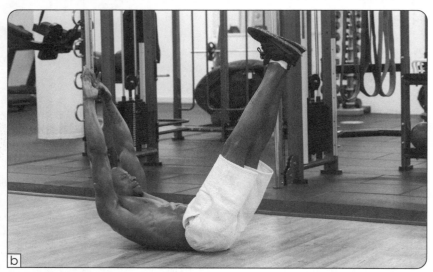

Performance

1. Simultaneously raise your legs and arms to reach vertical. As you do so, flex your spine to take you into a crunch.

2. Lower to the start, not quite returning all the way to the floor.

Tips for Success

Abdominal V-ups are easy to modify. To make them easier, do them with bent knees. Holding resistance in your hands and even attached to your legs will take them up a level.

15
AB MAT CRUNCH

Level: Foundational

Placing an abdominal mat in the arch of your lumbar spine could be the one simple but important upgrade your abdominal training needs. This pivot point for your spine to flex over allows you to load your abs through a greater range of motion. It also limits the amount of spinal flexion.

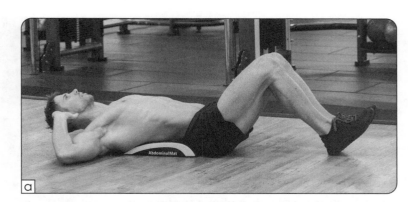

Setup

- Lie on the floor on your back as if ready to perform a basic crunch.
- Place the abdominal mat under your lower back, resting it in the groove of your lumbar area.
- The highest side of the abdominal mat should be closest to your hips.

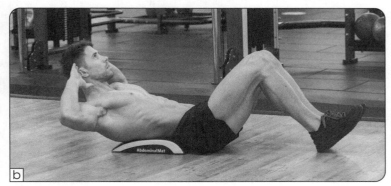

Performance

1. Begin to perform the basic crunch movement while keeping the abdominal mat firmly between the floor and your lower back.
2. Pull your ribs toward your pelvis as you flex your spine and contract your abs. The abdominal mat will intensify the contraction.
3. Return all the way down, taking your abdominals through a full range of motion as your spine extends over the abdominal mat.

Tips for Success

If you don't have access to an abdominal mat, use a small rolled-up towel. This can work almost as well and be used to mop your pool of sweat from the floor afterward!

16
DUMBBELL SERRATUS CRUNCH

Level: Intermediate

Dumbbell serratus crunches train your abdominals while activating your serratus anterior—muscles that are not just important for shoulder stability and health but also give a desirable look to your overall midsection when well developed.

Setup

- Lie on the floor as if to perform a basic crunch.
- Chest press two dumbbells to the roof.
- Bend your knees and hips to approximately 90 degrees, raising your feet off the floor.
- Keep your feet off the floor, legs static, and dumbbells held firmly in position throughout.

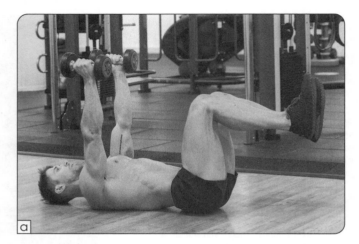

Performance

1. Contract your abdominals before initiating the crunch.
2. Press the dumbbells toward the roof using a crunchlike movement.
3. Keep your arms straight and vertical, allowing your shoulder blades to move freely.

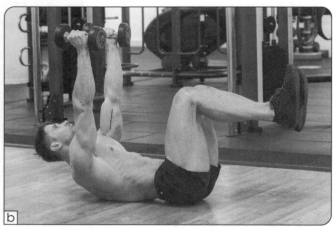

4. Reach the full crunch position before returning to the floor.

Tips for Success

Your serratus anterior is a muscle that looks like an extension of your abdominals and is located just above your obliques. Your serratus anterior also has an important role to play in shoulder stability and function, with long-term benefits to the health of your shoulders.

17
DEAD-BUG CRUNCH

Level: Intermediate

Dead bugs are an excellent core exercise that develop antirotational and antiextension strength. They can be combined with crunching movements to create the ultimate exercise for spinal health, performance, and aesthetics.

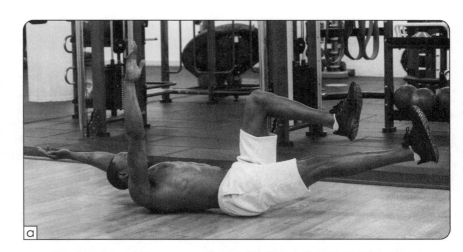

Setup

- Position yourself on your back.
- Reach your arms vertically toward the ceiling.
- Bend your hips and knees to 90 degrees, keeping your feet off the floor.
- Imagine pulling your lower back in toward the floor and bracing your abdominals hard: Imagine 360 degrees of air around your spine and contract your abdominals.

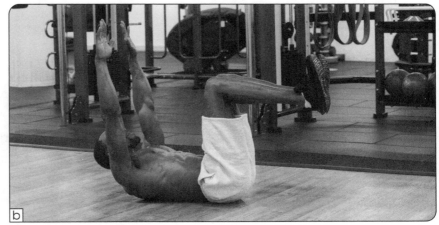

Performance

1. Begin to slowly lower one leg and the opposite arm overhead toward the floor.
2. Straighten your arm and leg fully, creating a long line through the opposite arm and leg.
3. Keep your core braced and resist rotation of your hips.
4. This is the end of the dead bug. Return to the start position.
5. Now, with your arms still vertical, perform a crunch.
6. Contract your abs hard to flex your spine.
7. Return to the start before repeating the sequence with the opposite arm and leg.

Tips for Success

You can add weight to your dead bugs by holding dumbbells in your hands and strapping small ankle weights to your legs.

18
HIGH-PULLEY CABLE CRUNCH ON STABILITY BALL

Level: Advanced

This exercise combines the stability ball with cable loading to create what may be one of the best six-pack builders of all time. It's essential that you're proficient at performing regular crunches on a stability ball before using this advanced variation.

Setup

- Fix a straight bar or dual-rope attachment to a cable pulley.
- Set your pulley cable to about two-thirds of its full height to start. Adjust the height from there depending on the feel of the exercise and the height of the stability ball.
- Position your stability ball just in front of the cables and sit on it.
- Make sure your position on the ball is stable, with your lower back resting on the highest part of the ball.
- As you extend over to reach for the cable, ensure you're far enough away to maintain tension in the cable.

Performance

1. Keep your arms straight and the cable overhead.
2. Contract your abdominals to begin the crunch movement.
3. As your spine flexes, engage your lats to pull the cable down toward your knees. Your elbows should still be straight.
4. If the cable is set high enough, the cable will remain safely overhead.
5. Tense your abs hard before returning to the start position, getting as much extension over the stability ball as possible.

Tips for Success

If you don't have access to a cable system, then using a resistance band at the same angle can work almost as well. This is a great at-home option.

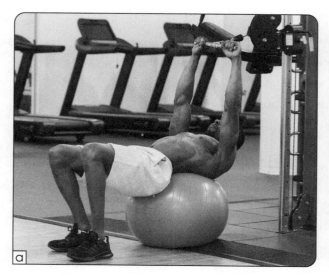
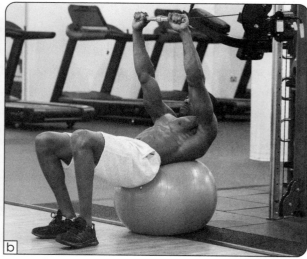

19
LOW-PULLEY CABLE CRUNCH

Level: Intermediate

Setting a cable system from a high angle loads your abdominals more in their fully shortened position. Here, setting up the cable from a lower height loads your abdominals more in their stretched position. Low-pulley cable crunches are notorious for next-day muscle soreness. You've been warned!

Setup

- Set your cable system low with a dual-rope attachment on the end of it.
- You may also use a stability ball, BOSU ball, or even abdominal mat for additional benefits.
- Position yourself far enough away from the cable that you can start and finish with a constant cable tension.
- Keep the rope over your shoulders throughout.

Performance

1. Pull your ribs down toward your pelvis as if executing a basic crunch.
2. The cable should be kept on your shoulders and will act to overload the crunch action.
3. After each crunch, return all the way to the start.
4. Exhale fully on the way up, and breathe in as you lower to the floor.

Tips for Success

Working your muscles at different lengths can emphasize different muscle growth mechanisms. Train at different muscle lengths to get the greatest results.

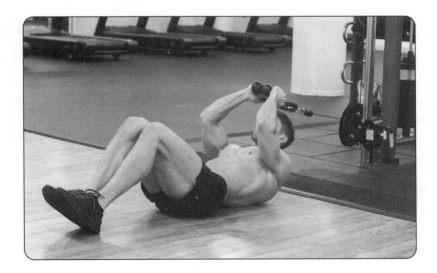

20
SICILIAN CRUNCH

Level: Advanced

Sicilian crunches overload your abdominals eccentrically. This is made possible by the change in the position of the resistance as you raise yourself and then lower. As you lower yourself with the resistance farther from your body, you're at a mechanical disadvantage. This creates an enhanced eccentric overload.

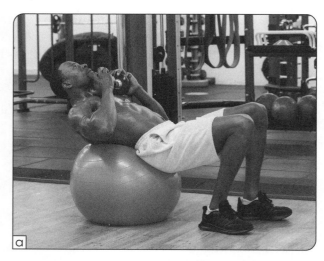

Setup

- Select your resistance. A dumbbell, plate, or medicine ball work equally well.
- Position yourself on the stability ball as if to perform a crunch.
- It will help if you use something to keep your feet firmly fixed to the floor, such as the underside of a bench, dumbbells on the floor, or a partner.

Performance

1. With the resistance close to your chest, begin to perform your crunch.
2. Here, you can choose to do a very isolated flexion of your spine or come a little higher into a partial sit-up.
3. When you reach the top of the crunch, press the resistance toward the ceiling. Hold it there.
4. Lower slowly, taking two to four seconds to return all the way down.
5. Fully stretch your abdominals before bringing the resistance back in and repeating.

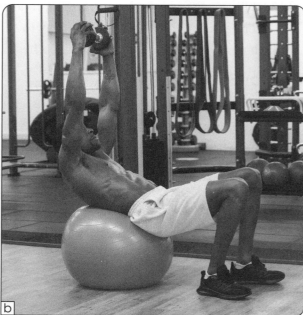

Tips for Success

Eccentric exercise is one of the most effective ways to cause a muscle to grow. This is because large amounts of mechanical tension and microtrauma occur during this phase of movement, activating a variety of mechanisms responsible for muscle hypertrophy.

21
OVERHEAD MEDICINE BALL SLAM

Level: Intermediate

Medicine ball slams are a good way to expose your abdominals to explosive training. This activates fast-twitch motor units and adds an element of athleticism to your workouts. Explosive training will become more important the older you get as these attributes naturally decline.

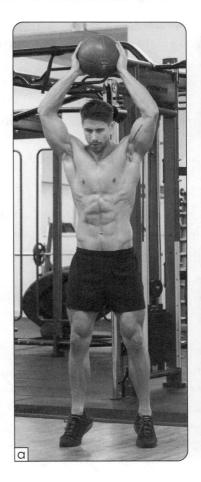
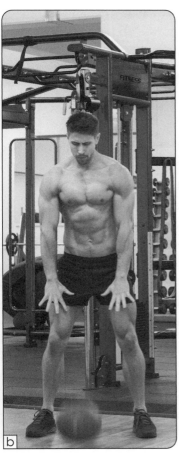

Setup

- Medicine ball slams can be done using a medicine ball that bounces or a dead ball. A ball that bounces will encourage a faster eccentric to concentric turnaround and more speed, whereas using a dead ball integrates more of a squatting movement to pick it back up off the floor each time. This is an important consideration and might affect the choice of flooring you do these on.
- Begin with the ball in hand and feet shoulder-width apart in an athletic position.

Performance

1. Raise the ball overhead, allowing your heels to leave the floor.
2. Pull the ball down; do not throw it. Think of this like performing a pull-down on a cable machine rather than a throw-in in a soccer match.
3. When you have pulled the ball almost all the way down, straighten your arms forcefully to throw the ball down as though driving it through the floor. Allow your chest to follow the ball and your spine to flex.
4. When using a dead ball, pick up the ball and repeat.
5. When using a ball with bounce, catch the ball at its highest point and then repeat another slam.

Tips for Success

Medicine ball throws can be used to train for both power and conditioning. For power development and recruitment of fast-twitch muscles, you want to minimize fatigue. Sets of no more than 10 reps work best so explosiveness can be maintained throughout. For conditioning purposes, you can use lighter medicine balls but for longer sets.

22

PLATE OVER KNEE CRUNCH

Level: Intermediate

These crunches combine a crunch with a reverse crunch. They effectively recruit both upper- and lower-abdominal fibers, and the plate adds load to the movement.

Setup

- Lie on the floor on your back as if ready to perform an ab crunch.
- Hold a plate overhead and hover your legs off the floor. Keep them from touching the floor throughout.
- Prevent your lower back from extending and lifting farther from the floor.

Performance

1. Simultaneously pull your knees toward your chest and chest toward your knees.
2. As you crunch to meet in the middle, pull the plate down toward your knees.
3. Reach the top of the crunch with your abdominals contracted as hard as possible.
4. Allow the plate to travel just over your knees.
5. Return to the start position. Do not let your legs or the plate return to the floor.

Tips for Success

Plate over knee crunches can be scaled down for beginners, too. Simply get rid of the plate, and as you reach the top of the crunch, use your hands to give your knees a hug. Once you can do 12 to 15 of these comfortably, try holding a very light Olympic plate or a water bottle.

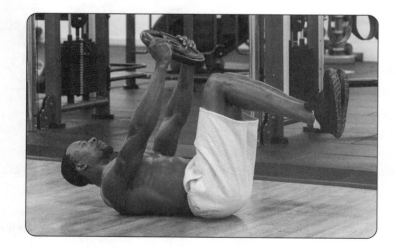

23
HEAVY BATTLE ROPE SLAM

Level: Intermediate

Heavy battle rope slams are a brilliant full-body conditioner used to shred your midsection. And by incorporating explosiveness into your routines, you'll recruit the often neglected fast-twitch muscle fibers of your abdominals. For abs that both look and perform well, heavy slams are a staple.

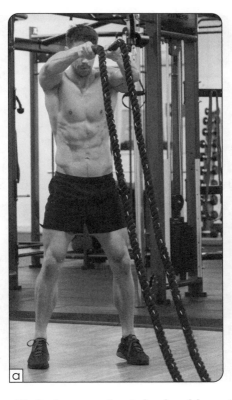
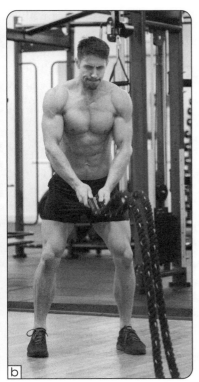

Setup

- Start with the battle ropes in an overhand grip and thumbs facing down the rope as opposed to facing toward you. People with shoulder issues might consider a grip with the thumbs facing more toward them.
- Begin in an athletic stance with feet approximately shoulder-width apart.

Performance

1. Keeping a tight hold of the rope, perform a triple extension of your ankles, knees, and hips to whip the rope upward.
2. Your arms should rise partially overhead but not fully.
3. When your hands and the rope reach the highest point, rapidly drive the rope down to the floor as hard as you can.
4. Reset and go again, making as much noise with the rope hitting the floor as possible. This will ensure maximal explosiveness throughout the set.

Tips for Success

The length and thickness of your battle ropes aren't often considered important, yet they are just as important as the weights you choose to pick up at the gym. If they are too thick or too long, your movements will be too slow or you'll risk shoulder injury. If they are too light or too short, the exercise won't be effective. Purchase wisely, or modify the length of your ropes accordingly.

24
AB WHEEL ROLLOUT WITH FLEXION

Level: Intermediate

Adding flexion to your ab wheel rollouts is a modification that recruits more of your abdominals. The additional flexion at the top activates more of your rectus abdominis, and as you lower, the antiextension nature of rollouts makes them an effective core builder.

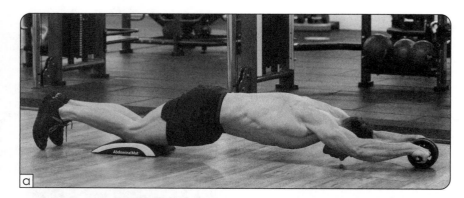

Setup

- You'll need an ab wheel and a foam pad or exercise mat for your knees (optional).
- Position yourself on all fours holding the ab wheel in front of you.
- Your knees should remain on the pad or mat throughout and act as a pivot point.

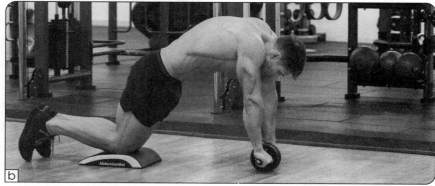

- Pinch your glutes together and brace your abs hard.

Performance

1. Push the ab roller forward, allowing your hips to drop with it.
2. Keep your abs and glutes engaged throughout to limit your lower back from sagging toward the floor. Excessive extension of your lumbar spine could cause pain or discomfort and should be closely monitored during rollouts.
3. Move the roller as far forward as you can. If you feel it in your lower back, then you've gone too far.
4. Resist extension of your lower back as you try to touch your nose to the floor.
5. To come back up, pull your arms down toward your hips, dragging the wheel toward you. Try to encourage maximal engagement of the lats here and, as always, the glutes and abs throughout.
6. As the roller reaches about the level of your shoulders, flex your spine as if to perform a crunch at the top.

Tips for Success

With modifications, ab wheel rollouts can be a useful exercise for beginners, too. Maintaining proper spinal and pelvic position as one rolls forward is commonly the hardest part of the exercise. To achieve this over time, practice in front of a wall, using the wall as a stopper and way to limit how far you drop. As you get better at these, move farther from the wall until the wall is no longer needed.

25
SEATED AB CABLE CRUNCH

Level: Intermediate

Seated ab cable crunches create a feeling like no crunch you've tried before. The intense contraction you get as your abdominals fully contract makes these a useful addition to any abdominal training routine.

Setup

- Use a dual-rope attachment on a single cable.
- Set a bench directly in front of and facing the cables.
- Set the cable high.
- Sit down and hold the cable close to your forehead.

Performance

1. Crunch down, pulling your rib cage toward the floor.
2. Your elbows may touch your knees.
3. Hold the bottom for a second, and squeeze your abs hard before coming back up.

Tips for Success

Seated ab cable crunches can be done facing toward the cables as shown or facing away from them. Facing toward them creates a more intense contraction toward the end of the crunch as you flex downward. When the cable comes from behind, the point of maximal load (due to leverage) is about midway through the crunch. You can experiment with both to see which works best.

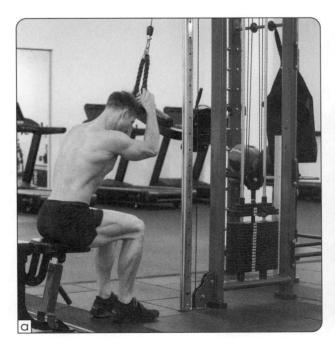
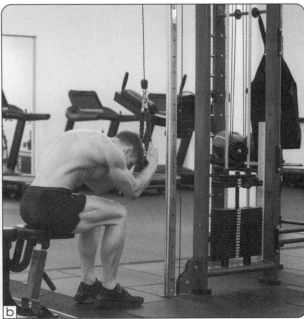

26
SEATED BAND CABLE CRUNCH

Level: Intermediate

Like seated ab cable crunches, these can be done using a band as well. The band can intensify the contraction as you crunch downward. This is an excellent exercise for awareness and feeling your abs work.

Setup

- Use a moderate-strength resistance band attached high. A power rack at the gym or secure beam in your home garage are good options.
- Set a bench or chair directly in front of and facing where the band is attached.
- Sit down and hold the band close to your forehead.

Performance

1. Keeping the band close to your forehead, crunch down, pulling your rib cage toward the floor.
2. Your elbows may touch your knees.
3. Hold the bottom for a second and squeeze your abs hard before coming back up.
4. Do not let the band fire you back up too fast.

Tips for Success

- Combine these with a brutal ab drop set using two bands.
- Hold two lighter bands instead of one.
- Once you reach near failure, release one band, and continue to do the crunches with the remaining band. Good luck!

27
STICK CRUNCH

Level: Intermediate

Stick crunches show a combination of core and abdominal strength and hip mobility. As a novel way to perform crunches and for an extra challenge, do these with either a wooden dowel or long resistance band held in both hands.

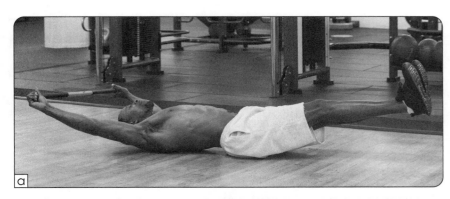

Setup

- Lie on the floor with your legs straight and arms fully overhead.
- Hold the wooden dowel with hands approximately shoulder-width apart or a little wider.
- One full repetition is when you return to this position.

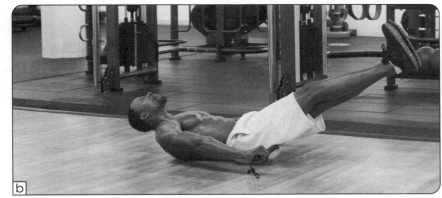

Performance

1. At the same time, lift the dowel and your feet off the floor.
2. Come up into a crunch, pulling your knees in toward your chest while bringing the dowel toward the middle.
3. At the highest point in the crunch (somewhat of a sit-up), attempt to take the dowel over your feet.
4. Take the dowel under your legs and return flat on the floor. The dowel will rest somewhere between your hamstrings and the floor.
5. Reverse the motion and come up into the crunch, but this time attempt to take the dowel in the opposite direction and back over your feet.
6. Return to lying flat on the floor with the dowel overhead.

Tips for Success

The first time you try stick crunches don't wear shoes. Even the half-inch (1.3 cm) sole of your sneakers can be enough to stop you from getting the dowel over your feet. As your mobility improves, you can put your sneakers back on and try again.

28

BUTT SCRATCHER

Level: Intermediate

The drag movement in butt scratchers makes these effective at working your abdominals through both spinal flexion *and* posterior pelvic tilt. This double attack on your abs works them hard in their fully shortened position.

Setup

- Begin sitting upright with your hands on the floor. If you find your arms aren't long enough to do these, place your hands on yoga blocks or push-up handles.
- Place your heels on a pair of core sliders.
- Push through your hands to raise your butt off the floor.

Performance

1. Ensuring your butt stays off the floor throughout, keep your knees straight and begin to pull the core sliders toward you.
2. Bring the sliders as far in as possible, allowing your pelvis to tilt under and travel almost behind you.
3. Your butt is still not touching the floor and should be as far off the floor as your arm length allows.
4. Your abdominals should be firing like crazy. If they're not, give them some help by tensing as hard as you can. Hold for a split second.
5. Slide back to the start position.

Tips for Success

If you don't have access to purpose-built core sliders, don't worry. Butt scratchers and other core-slider exercises can work equally well using a pair of low-cost furniture sliders, old magazines, or even paper plates on a rug.

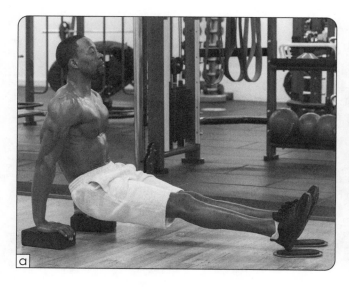
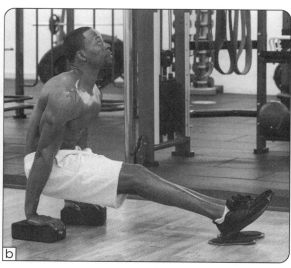

Chapter 8

Targeting Your Lower Abs

For many people, the lower area of the abdominals can be a trouble spot. Facing stubborn belly fat and muscles that just will not grow can be frustrating—especially if you're training hard and trying to eat right. Having a low level of body fat will allow you to see four- or even six-pack abs. But to achieve the fabled eight-pack, specific exercises that target the lower portion of your abdominals need to be done.

The ability to isolate a certain area of your abdominals does not exist. Even if your goal is to isolate the rectus abdominis muscle as a whole, it is still impossible to do that without activating other muscles at the same time (for example your external obliques). However, with the right exercises and techniques, it is possible to emphasize the muscle fibers that make up the lower portion of your rectus abdominis.

In chapter 2, we covered abdominal anatomy. As a quick refresher, you'll remember that the rectus abdominis extends the length of the abdomen, from the pubis to the sternum and three ribs. To work the muscle fully, you need to use exercises that align you correctly and pull your lower ribs and pubis closer together. The lower abdominals are largely responsible for the action of pulling the pelvis upward (posterior pelvic tilt), while the middle and upper abdominal fibers are responsible for pulling your ribs down (spinal flexion).

To work your lower abdominals most efficiently, exercises that involve a posterior tilt of your pelvis are best. The following exercises will get closer to your goal of having six-pack abs.

1
BASIC REVERSE CRUNCH

Level: Foundational

Basic reverse crunches are a foundational exercise to teach lower-abdominal activation. The simplicity of the exercise provides the best environment in which to focus on the correct technique for working your lower abdominals. Unless you can perform basic reverse crunches, you will not get the most out of the other exercises featured in this chapter. Pay close attention to the execution of the performance steps, and don't underestimate the effectiveness of this simple ab exercise.

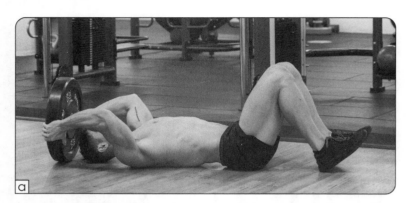

Setup

- Lie on the floor on your back. You can lie on a mat (optional).
- Bend your knees approximately 90 degrees, and place your feet flat on the floor.
- Use a medicine ball, weight, or sturdy support held overhead as you reverse crunch.

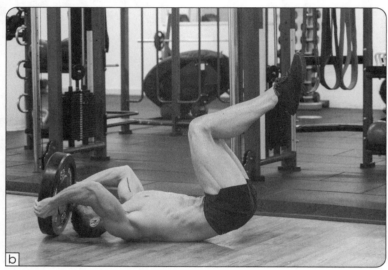

Performance

1. Take a deep breath in and contract your abdominals.
2. Initiate by first thinking "pelvis to ribs," followed by your knees coming up toward your chest.
3. Exhale fully and squeeze your abs as hard as you can when you reach the top.
4. Lower your feet toward the floor at a controlled speed, keeping tension in your midsection throughout.
5. You can tap the floor gently (without creating momentum), or you can keep your feet off the floor for the duration.
6. Focus on tension and feeling it, and don't worry about how many repetitions you're doing. If you don't feel these in your abdominals, then you're not doing them right.

Tips for Success

- To make reverse crunches harder, perform them with slightly straighter knees.
- To make them easier, tuck your knees in closer.
- More advanced reverse crunch variations are featured later in this chapter.

2
LEG RAISE

Level: Intermediate

Reverse crunches require a bent-knee position. Because of a longer lever arm length, leg raises with your legs extended are more difficult than reverse crunches. For that reason, leg raises are one of the best ways to progress reverse crunches without requiring extra equipment.

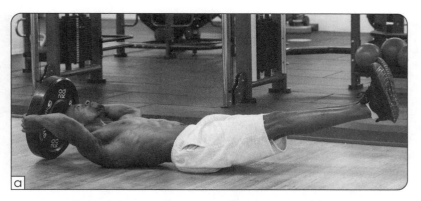

Setup

- Lie on your back on the floor. You can use a mat (optional).
- Use a medicine ball, weight, or immovable support held overhead.
- Start with your head down and feet hovering slightly off the floor.
- Your knees should be straight but not locked.
- Your lower back should be pushed toward the floor to limit hyperextension of the lumbar spine.

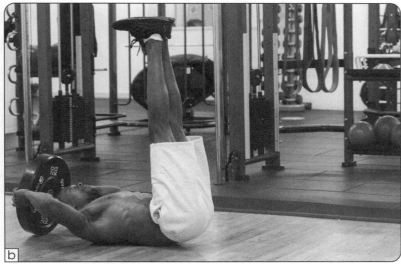

- Some people find leg raises off the floor to be more comfortable with a very small rolled-up towel under their lower back.

Performance

1. Contract your abdominals to initiate a pull from your pelvis.
2. Raise your legs up and toward vertical.
3. Raise them until your pelvis tilts at the top of the movement. This is when hip flexion stops and the posterior tilt begins.
4. Exhale fully at the top.
5. Lower under control, maintaining abdominal tension without letting your heels touch the floor.
6. Do not use momentum to raise your legs. If this happens, then you can add a brief pause at the bottom of each repetition.

Tips for Success

- The most effective portion of the leg raise is at the top where your pelvis begins to tilt. Doing them flat on the floor can cause a slight drop in abdominal tension at the top caused by gravity.
- To overcome a drop in tension at the top of leg raises and as a progression, use a decline bench.

3
ECCENTRIC LEG RAISE

Level: Advanced

Eccentric leg raises work by manipulating lever arm length: You resist more as you lower the legs to the floor (eccentric—longer lever arm) than when you raise the legs (concentric—shorter lever arm). Because eccentric exercises are a highly effective technique for building muscle on any body part, your abdominals can benefit from this method as well. You could see these as a reverse crunch on the way up, and a leg raise on the way down. If you're more advanced, then you have the option to weight these, too. See the Tips for Success section for more information on adding weight.

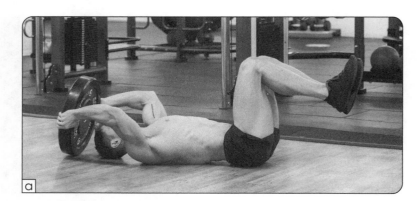

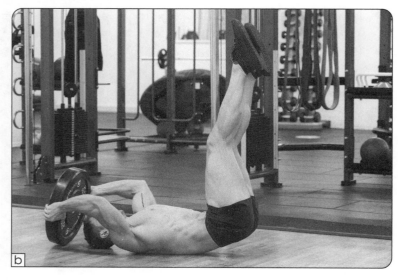

Setup

- Lie on the floor on your back. You can use a mat (optional).
- Use a medicine ball, heavy weight, or sturdy support overhead that you can grab.
- Your head is down, core engaged, and lower back pressed toward the floor.
- Your knees should be bent to about 90 degrees.
- Keep your feet approximately an inch (2.5 cm) off the floor throughout the performance.

Performance

1. Initiate a knee raise by first thinking "pelvis to ribs," followed by raising your knees toward your chest.
2. Bring your knees as high as you can until your hips come off the floor as your pelvis tilts.
3. When you reach the highest point, straighten your legs. This should now look like a leg raise.
4. Keep your legs straight and lower them under control in about four seconds, exhaling as you do so as this requires the greatest effort.
5. Bend your knees at the bottom and repeat, inhaling on the lift upwards.

Tips for Success

If you're more advanced, you have the option to overload the eccentric portion of these leg raises even more. The best way to do this would be using a few pounds of weight strapped around your ankles.

4
DECLINE REVERSE CRUNCH

Level: Intermediate

The most important part of a reverse crunch is at the top of the movement. This is where the lower fibers of your rectus abdominis work to create the posterior pelvic tilt we've spoken of before. Unfortunately, because of leverage factors, reverse crunches off the floor or a flat surface mean that you lose abdominal tension at the top of the movement. The solution is to do them using a slight decline. Decline angles from 10- to 45-degrees will work.

Setup

- Set a bench to a decline. The greater the decline, the more the difficult the exercise.
- Position yourself on the bench with your legs in the direction of the decline.
- Hold on to the bench overhead.

Performance

1. Holding firmly overhead so you don't move or slide down the bench, pull your knees in toward your chest.
2. Your knees will remain approximately 90 degrees throughout.
3. Imagine pulling your pelvis toward your rib cage as much as possible and your hips coming off the bench at the top.
4. Squeeze your abs hard at the top before lowering fully under control.
5. Do not let your feet touch the floor between repetitions.

Tips for Success

- Although you might consider a steeper decline to be better (for example, 45 degrees being better than 10 degrees), there are other factors to consider.
- For most, a 30-degree decline works best for both comfort and optimizing abdominal tension.

5

DECLINE MEDICINE BALL REVERSE CRUNCH

Level: Advanced

There are many ways to progress and add weight to reverse crunches. One of the most efficient ways is to use a medicine ball between your knees. If the ball becomes too heavy, it's easily released midset so you can keep going and maintain abdominal tension. Clenching a ball between your knees activates your adductor muscles too, which can benefit your overall core stability.

Setup

- Set a bench to a decline. The greater the decline, the more difficult the exercise.
- Position yourself on the bench with your legs in the direction of the decline.
- Hold on to the bench overhead, or use any grip your bench might have.
- Clench a medicine ball between your knees.

Performance

1. Holding on to the bench firmly so you don't move or slide down, pull your knees in toward your chest, bringing the medicine ball with it.
2. Your knees will remain approximately 90 degrees throughout.
3. Imagine pulling your pelvis toward your rib cage as much as possible, and your hips come off the bench at the top.
4. Squeeze your abs hard at the top before lowering fully.
5. Do not let your feet touch the bench or floor between repetitions.

Tips for Success

For an abdominal intensity method then try this drop-set:
Begin with a heavier medicine ball, then once you are near failure, switch it for a lighter ball or even body weight. Your abs won't know what hit them!

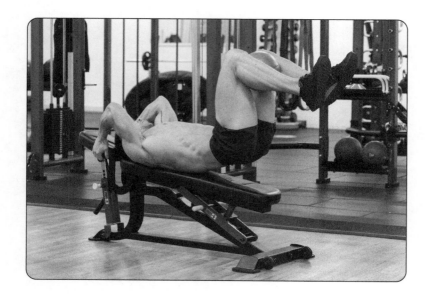

6

HAMSTRING-ACTIVATED REVERSE CRUNCH

Level: Advanced

Your abdominals do not act as hip flexors. For that reason, as you flex your hips during a reverse crunch or leg raise, only a small portion of the exercise will work your abs the hardest. By activating your hamstrings, you can partially stop your hip flexors from doing most of the exercise, increasing activation of your abdominals. This is an advanced technique and not to be done unless you have mastered basic reverse crunches.

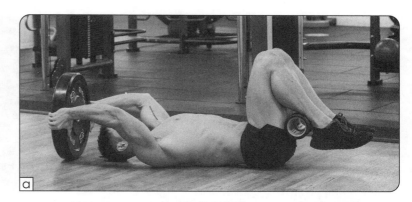

Setup

- Assume the basic reverse crunch position.
- Place a foam roller behind your knees, clenched between your calves and hamstrings.
- Squeeze the foam roller hard throughout by activating your hamstrings.
- You may also use a thick rolled-up towel.

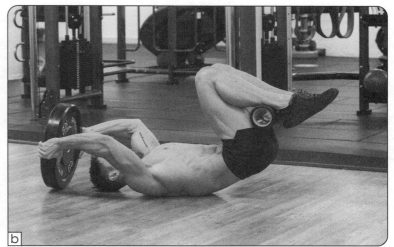

Performance

1. Initiate the exercise by thinking "pelvis to ribs," followed by your knees coming up toward your chest.
2. Squeeze the foam roller firmly to hold it in place.
3. Exhale fully at the top and contract your abs hard.
4. Lower your feet toward the floor, keeping tension in your midsection.
5. The foam roller should still be in position and squeezed hard.
6. Do not touch the floor with your feet.

Tips for Success

You don't have to use a foam roller for hamstring-activated reverse crunches. In fact, anything you can comfortably squeeze between your calves and hamstrings will work. This can include a basketball, soccer ball, or even rolled-up piece of clothing for at-home use.

7
REVERSE CRUNCH DEAD-BUG COMBO

Level: Intermediate

The reverse crunch dead-bug combo uses a basic reverse crunch combined with a dead bug to provide the benefits of both exercises in one move. Dead bugs are one of the most effective exercises for developing core stability in an anti-rotational and antiextension capacity, while reverse crunches do exactly what you want in hitting those lower abdominal fibers. Use the combination of these two exercises to develop a strong and chiseled midsection and healthy back.

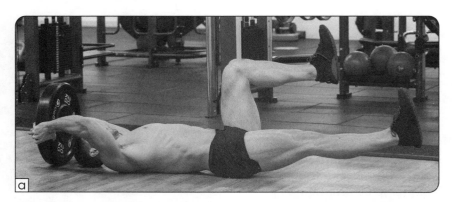

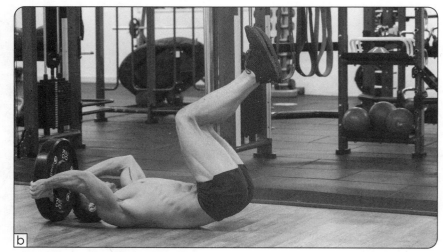

Setup

- Start on the floor, lying on your back.
- Raise both feet off the floor so your knees and hips are bent approximately 90 degrees.
- Press your lower back into the floor to activate your core.
- Hold a heavy object overhead to keep you in position. A kettlebell or weight plate is best.

Performance

1. Returning to the setup position every time, begin by extending one leg so it's as long as possible. Do not let your heel touch the floor.
2. At the same time, extend the opposite hand as far overhead as possible. This will require you to let go of the overhead weight with that hand.
3. The opposite arm and leg should be as far from one another as possible, and the other arm and leg are in the original position.
4. Repeat with the opposite arm and leg. This is your dead bug.
5. Keeping hold of the weight overhead, lift your pelvis off the floor into a partial reverse crunch—a reverse crunch without lowering all the way to the floor.
6. Lower your hips, returning to the setup position.
7. Repeat with a dead bug on each side followed by a partial reverse crunch.

Tips for Success

- You can progress the reverse crunch dead-bug combo by using small ankle weights strapped to your ankles and even wrists.
- Lower your legs with bent knees for an easier version, or keep your legs straight throughout to take it up a level.

8
STABILITY BALL KNEE TUCK

Level: Intermediate

Stability ball knee tucks are often avoided out of fear of looking awkward. When you get them right, though, they not only help your abs look good but also do a world of good for your whole-body balance and stability. Take your time with these, get the setup right, and don't rush your reps.

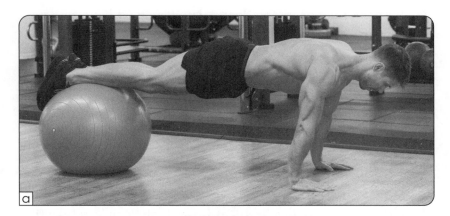

Setup

- With your hands on the floor in a position similar to a plank, place your feet on top of a stability ball.
- Your shins are in contact with the ball.
- Engage your core and maintain stability.
- This is your start and finish position.

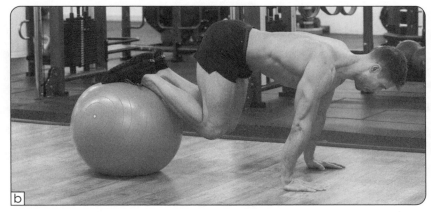

Performance

1. Pull your knees in toward your chest, allowing the ball to roll down your shins.
2. Bring your knees just beyond level with your hips to maximize the tuck of your pelvis.
3. Keep your shoulders firmly stacked over your elbows and wrists.
4. Return to the start.
5. Do not perform these too fast, and ensure you stay on the center of the ball.

Tips for Success

If you have good balance and core strength, you may find stability ball knee tucks too easy. If this is the case then you can try pikes using the stability ball instead: Keep your knees straight and push your hips up to create an inverted V with your body.

9

SUSPENSION KNEE TUCK

Level: Intermediate

Suspension knee tucks are a good way to improve core stability and develop your lower abs. Using a suspension trainer is more stable than the more traditional knee tucks using a stability ball. For that reason, they are more suitable for beginners or if you struggle with balance. Don't underestimate them, though. Done correctly, these will give your abs the workout they need.

Setup

- Place your feet inside the stirrup or handle of the suspension trainer.
- With your hands on the floor, assume a planklike position.
- Engage your core and maintain stability.
- This is your start and finish position.

Performance

1. Pull your knees up toward your chest.
2. Contract your abdominals and tuck your knees toward your chest as far as you can. A little spine flexion is fine here.
3. Return to the start position, making yourself as long as possible.
4. Keep your lower back from caving or hips dropping too far.
5. Exhale as you pull your knees in, and inhale as you take them back.

Tips for Success

The farther your hands are from the hanging point of the suspension trainer at the start, the harder the knee tuck is.

10
PIKE ON A ROWING MACHINE

Level: Advanced

The rowing machine offers an unconventional opportunity to perform various abdominal exercises such as pikes and knee tucks. The seat of the rower slides with ease, and as you pike your hips up, there is even an increased resistance as the seat travels somewhat up hill. This is true for most popular rowers.

Setup

- Place your feet on top of the seat of the rowing machine.
- Your hands are on the floor and head faces away from the front of the rower.
- Begin in a planklike position with your spine neutral and core engaged.
- This is your start and finish position.

Performance

1. Pike your hips up by pushing them toward the ceiling.
2. Pull your feet toward your upper body by sliding the seat of the rower.
3. The top position is when your pelvis tilts or you've reached the highest point you can.
4. Exhale fully and contract your abs hard at the top.
5. Return to the start, lowering until your hips are fully straight.
6. Resist letting the seat slide back too fast as you lower yourself.

Tips for Success

- Adding progression to pikes isn't as easy as it is in some other abdominal exercises. You can add more reps over time, but this becomes ineffective at some point. And there's no easy way to add weight.
- To make pikes harder, try adding strategic pauses throughout the movement. Taking a two-second pause at the top of each rep can significantly increase the challenge.
- You may also slow your repetitions and focus on time under tension.

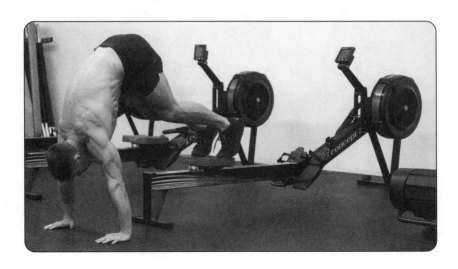

11
SUSPENSION PIKE

Level: Advanced

One of the most effective ways to perform pikes is by using a suspension trainer. It provides a small amount of instability, especially in the sideways direction but not so much that it becomes awkward. If you struggle with balance when using a stability ball, then pikes using a suspension trainer can be equally effective and a more appealing prospect for most people.

Setup

- Place your feet inside the stirrup or handles of the suspension trainer.
- With your hands on the floor, assume a planklike position.
- Engage your core and maintain stability.
- This is your start and finish position.

Performance

1. Pike your hips up by pushing them toward the ceiling.
2. Pull your feet toward your upper body by pulling the suspension trainer toward your hands.
3. The top position is when your hips have risen to the highest point you can attain.
4. Exhale fully at the top and squeeze your abs as hard as you can.
5. Lower under control, and return all the way to the start.

Tips for Success

- To make pikes harder, you can manipulate repetition speed.
- Try adding slow eccentric contractions, pauses, or extra pulses at the top of each repetition for more intensity.

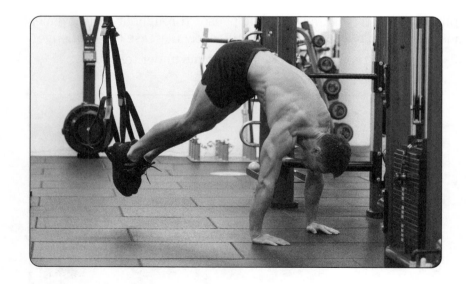

12
SLIDER KNEE TUCK

Level: Intermediate

Slider knee tucks use core sliders to achieve the knee tuck position. Resistance is provided by the friction of the sliders on the floor. Using sliders can create more stability than when doing the same exercise on either a stability ball or suspension trainer, making these a useful variation if your balance is limited.

Setup

- Begin in a planklike position.
- Place your feet firmly in the middle of each core slider.
- The flooring must be suitable for the sliders to travel on.

Performance

1. Pull the sliders across the floor toward your hands.
2. Pull your knee in toward your chest as far as you can.
3. The top position is when your knees are closest to your chest, your pelvis is slightly rotated (posterior tilt), and you maintain abdominal tension.
4. Exhale as you come to the top, and inhale as you lower.
5. Return all the way to the starting position.
6. Do not allow your back to cave toward the floor or hips to drop too far.

Tips for Success

- Hockey slide trainers are another useful way to perform these.
- If no equipment is available, then placing your feet on paper plates allows them to slide along the floor.

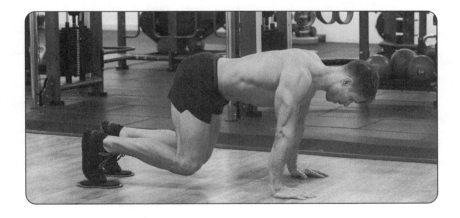

13
LOW-PULLEY KNEE IN

Level: Advanced

The low-pulley knee in is an extremely useful exercise that is often forgotten about. While these do look similar to reverse crunches and work in much the same way, positioning a cable in the way shown allows a gradual and progressive overload.

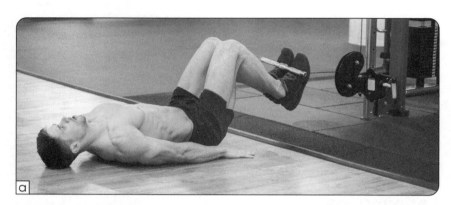

Setup

- Set a cable to its lowest height and attach a straight bar.
- Lie on your back on the floor with feet facing toward the cables.
- Ensure you have enough distance from the cables to straighten your legs.
- Mimic a basic reverse crunch position with knees and hips bent to about 90 degrees.

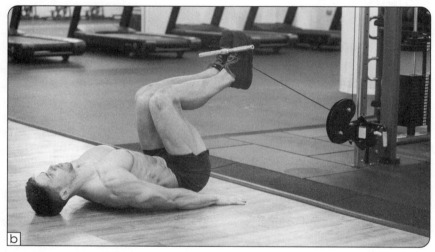

- Keep your ankles flexed upward (dorsiflexed) and hook the straight bar onto your toes.

Performance

1. Pull your knees up toward your chest.
2. The straight bar should remain hooked on your feet and load the movement.
3. When your knees have been brought in fully and your hips are off the floor, hold this for a brief second to feel the tension through your entire midsection.
4. Fight the weight and lower to the start.
5. The movement is very short, and you should lower only to a point where you can still keep the straight bar and cable hooked on your feet.
6. This exercise may take some getting used to, but the effort is worth it.

Tips for Success

If available, use the micro cable weights that quite often go unused. These are weights that give you a small increment in load and can be added to the cable stack.

14
BANDED LYING LEG RAISE

Level: Intermediate

The banded lying leg raise is a regular leg raise with your back on the floor combined with the instability of gripping a shaky band. The leg raise works by taking you into the posteriorly tilted position that's required for lower-ab development, while the band offers multiple advantages, adds complexity, and challenges your entire core in an unstable manner.

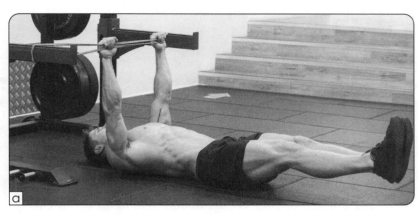

Setup

- Loop a resistance band between two sturdy supports, such as a power rack.
- Make sure there's no slack in the band, and set it about hip height to start.
- Lie on your back under the band. You should be able to reach up and grab it.
- Hold the band at arm's length and level with your chest.

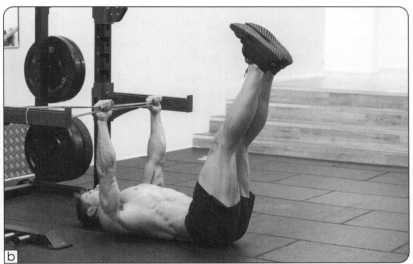

Performance

1. Attempt to pull the band down by engaging your lats. This will somewhat resemble a straight-arm lat pull-down motion.
2. Press your lower back toward the floor, contract your abdominals, and raise your legs as if to perform a leg raise.
3. The band might cause you to shake. This is normal and part of the challenge.
4. Raise your legs to the point that your hips just leave the floor.
5. Keep your lats engaged throughout by pulling the band down.
6. Lower your legs toward the floor, but do not allow your heels to touch it.
7. Exhale on the leg raise, and take a deep breath in as you lower.

Tips for Success

- If the focus of this exercise is abdominal activation, then a higher-strength resistance band is best. But if you want the benefits of using an unstable environment, then a lighter resistance band is more unstable.
- More band resistance is not necessarily better, and you should choose resistance based on your core and abdominal training priorities.

15
PLATE HANGING KNEE RAISE

Level: Advanced

Hanging knee raises are a staple exercise for eight-pack abs. They are one of the most commonly used exercises to target the lower portion of your rectus abdominis. However, it can sometimes be difficult to add weight when they become too easy. Besides purchasing your own ankle weights or awkwardly holding something between your knees or feet, you can also use equipment found at most gyms to add considerable weight. Because the weight is directly on your thighs, you will get very little assistance from other muscles outside of your lower abs, too. All you need is a dipping belt and a weight plate.

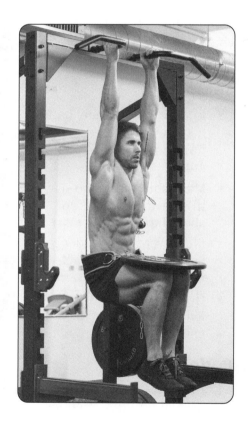

Setup

- Put a dipping belt on according to its intended use.
- Start with a light weight.
- Shorten the chain enough that the bottom of the plate does not hang lower than your knees. This will depend on the size of the plate used and the design of the dipping belt.
- Start in a hanging knee raise position, either hanging on a bar, using an abdominal sling, or using a captain's chair bench.

Performance

1. Keep the plate flat against your thighs as you raise your knees toward your chest.
2. The dipping belt enables the plate to stay close to your thighs throughout.
3. The highest point is when your knees rise past the level of your hips and your pelvis posteriorly tilts.
4. Do not use this weighted variation unless you have first mastered a knee raise with body weight only.

Tips for Success

Plate hanging knee raises can be done hanging off a bar, in a captain's chair, or even holding on to a dipping bar.

16
GARHAMMER LEG RAISE

Level: Advanced

The Garhammer leg raise and its variations are great exercises for hitting the lower portion of your rectus abdominis and working it hard in its active range of motion (through posterior pelvic tilt). Garhammer leg raises were invented by sports scientist John Garhammer, PhD, and are a popular exercise in strength and conditioning circles.

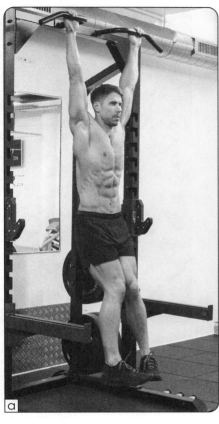
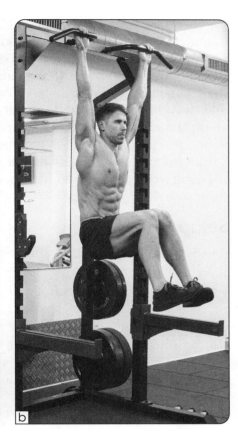

Setup

- Jump up to a bar and grab it using an overhand grip.
- Use a grip width most comfortable for you.
- Keep your shoulders strong and away from your ears.
- Your toes should point toward each other, and your heels face slightly outward.
- Your knees should face inward and remain at this angle throughout.

Performance

1. Initiate by contracting your abdominals hard before the movement takes place.
2. Do not swing or use momentum.
3. Imagine pulling your pelvis up toward your ribs as your legs raise.
4. Your knees should have a slight bend in them, and your toes remain pointed at each other.
5. Rise to a point just past thighs parallel to the floor.
6. Lower under control, maintaining abdominal tension.
7. Lower only two-thirds of the way, and avoid returning to the full hanging start.

Tips for Success

- As a progression, perform Garhammer raises with knees straighter.
- As a regression, do Garhammer raises on a bench, using a slight decline.

17
SEATED RACK TOES TO BAR

Level: Hardcore

The seated rack toes to bar is an unconventional take on the more popular hanging toes to bar. Unlike the hanging toes to bar that tends to be done using a lot of momentum and very little abdominal engagement, the rack toes to bar puts you in an ideal position to get maximum output from your lower abs. Once you try them, you'll understand why they work so well.

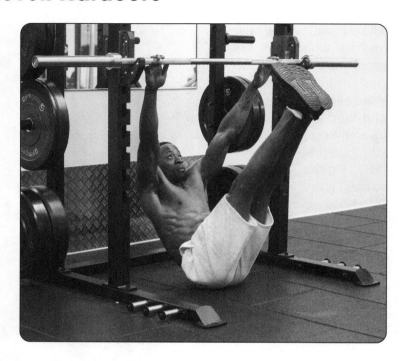

Setup

- Set a bar in a rack approximately hip height or higher.
- When you sit on the floor, you should be able to grab hold of the bar from under it.
- While gripping the bar, lean slightly back.
- Start and finish with your heels off the floor.

Performance

1. Pull down on the bar as if to perform a straight-arm lat pull-down. This will engage your lats and your abdominals further.
2. Raise your legs up toward the bar.
3. Attempt to touch the bar with your toes or shins before lowering.
4. Do not let your heels touch the floor.
5. Do not use momentum.

Tips for Success

- By engaging your lats in the pulling-down motion, there's an even greater benefit to your core. Not only will your lower abs get a great workout, but so will the rest of your midsection.
- The seated rack toes to bar has an excellent transfer to the hanging toes to bar, eventually allowing you to do them without cheating or using momentum.

18
HANGING TOES TO BAR

Level: Hardcore

The hanging toes to bar is a self-limiting exercise, meaning that to be able to do it correctly, you have to touch your toes to the bar each and every time. Ideally, for the purpose of developing your abs, this should be done without momentum. The hanging toes to bar is often used in conditioning-style workouts where excessive swinging is involved. This might enable you to achieve the most reps, but it will not do much for your lower abs.

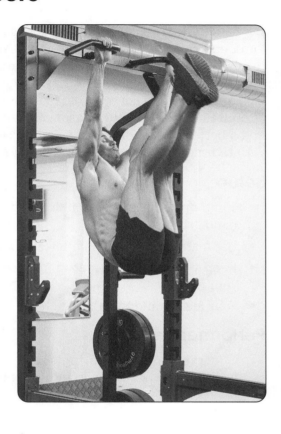

Setup

- Jump up to a bar and grab it using an overhand grip.
- Use a grip width most comfortable for you.
- Keep your shoulders strong and away from your ears.
- Your legs are hanging and core is engaged.

Performance

1. Contract your abdominals and imagine pushing your lower back into an imaginary hand placed behind it or a real hand if you have a partner.
2. Pull your pelvis up toward your ribs and begin to raise your legs.
3. Never swing or use momentum.
4. Keep your knees extended, with only a very slight bend.
5. *Note:* The goal is to work your abdominals, not merely to get your toes to the bar for performance reasons.
6. Raise your legs to a point where you can touch your toes or shins to the bar. If you cannot, then just short of this is acceptable.
7. Lower under control and attempt to come to a dead halt between each repetition to avoid the swing.

Tips for Success

When training your abdominals, your lack of grip strength should never hold you back. To help this try using weightlifting straps or similar to get a better grip for a more targeted abs exercise.

19

BAR HANGING LEG RAISE

Level: Advanced

Bar hanging leg raises are a staple exercise for your lower-abdominal region. The aim of this exercise is to raise your legs to a point where they are approximately parallel with the floor. Unlike the toes to bar exercise, you're not required to raise your feet as high as the bar. For this reason, it's easier to do and a better option for either beginners or those with tightness that might limit range of motion.

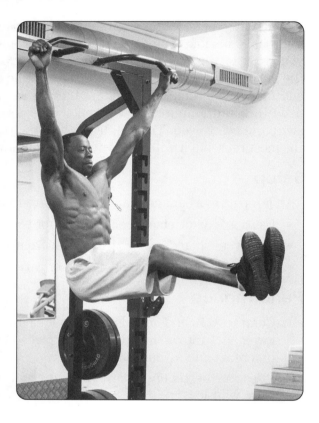

Setup

- Jump up to a bar and grab it using an overhand grip.
- Use a grip width most comfortable for you.
- Keep your shoulders strong and away from your ears.
- Your feet should remain together.

Performance

1. Contract your abdominals and imagine pushing your lower back into an imaginary hand placed on it or a real hand if you have a partner.
2. Pull your pelvis up toward your ribs and begin to raise your legs.
3. Do not use momentum.
4. Keep your knees extended with only a slight bend.
5. Raise your legs to a point just past parallel to the floor.
6. Lower under control, attempting to come to a dead halt between each repetition to avoid swinging.

Tips for Success

There are many movements you can add to hanging leg raises as a way to mix up your abdominal training. For example, you can try bicycling your legs, raising one leg at a time, flutter kicks, or even raising your knees in a froglike position.

20
KNEE RAISE ON DIPPING BAR

Level: Advanced

Inspired by the movements of Olympic gymnasts and their impressive feats of core strength, dipping bars, like parallel bars, can be used for a variety of exercises. Performing knee raises from this position has a different feel than hanging on a bar. There is little requirement for gripping a bar, and some people find that momentum is easier to control.

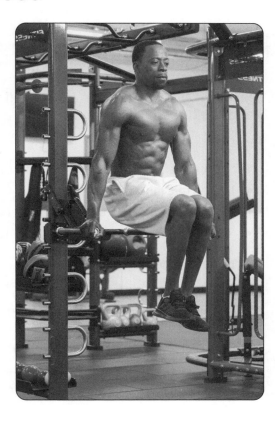

Setup

- Jump up to a dipping bar and hold there with your elbows fully straight but not hyperextended.
- Do not swing or lose stability.

Performance

1. Contract your abdominals and raise your knees up toward your chest.
2. Do not swing and do not use momentum; let your abs do the lifting!
3. Push your pelvis back slightly as you rise. This will further help the posterior tilt of the pelvis at the top.
4. Lower to the start under control.

Tips for Success

- Include static holds at the top of your knee raises for gymnastics-inspired core strength.
- You can also try static holds with straight legs if you're up for the challenge.

21
ELEVATED STABILITY BALL KNEE TUCK

Level: Advanced

Elevated stability ball knee tucks require a little setup, but once you're in position, you'll realize the benefits. These are sure to become one of your new favorite exercises. Doing knee tucks on a stability ball with elevation requires good overall core strength and stability. Elevating your elbows to the same height as the ball is much easier on your upper body than having your hands on the floor. This helps shift the focus to hitting your abs hard rather than to upper-body strength or cranky shoulders that are getting in the way.

Setup

- Start with a box or high step and a stability ball. Both should be approximately the same height.
- Place your elbows on the box.
- Position your shins on the stability ball.
- Squeeze your glutes and engage your core.

Performance

1. Pull your knees up toward the box.
2. Maintain side-to-side stability while dragging the stability ball up toward the box in a straight line.
3. Contract your abdominals hard at the top as you exhale fully.
4. Reverse back to the start position by pushing the stability ball away from the box.
5. Always return to a strong and stable start position in which your glutes and abs are maximally engaged.

Tips for Success

If you have shoulder issues, then regular stability ball pikes and knee tucks can be painful. Positioning your elbows on a box might help you prevent the pain, and it works your abs harder.

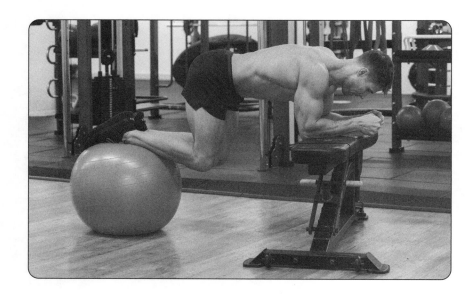

Targeting Your Obliques

Chapter 2 covered abdominal anatomy and how the external obliques form part of the lateral abdominal wall alongside your internal obliques and transverse abdominis (TVA). Your external obliques are more important visually as they taper down the side of your waist to complement your six-pack abs. Developing impressive obliques requires lateral flexion and rotational movements. These can include the use of bands and cables that offer constant tension or medicine balls that allow for explosive movement.

The rotational and lateral flexion exercises that activate your obliques were described in chapter 3. Crunches and sit-ups with twisting motions are common exercises for your obliques. However, exercises like rollouts, pikes, and knee raises have the potential to activate them even more. Even pull-ups have the potential to activate them to a large degree. It's therefore evident that twisting crunches and sit-up motions aren't necessary to train your obliques, but they can be useful additions to complement some of the other exercises you're already doing. This chapter covers the twisting crunch and sit-up motions you should include in your training for a complete set of abs.

Chapter 3 also discussed chopping motions, which usually twist from an upright position (e.g., standing, split, half kneeling). Exercises that contain chopping motions are considered a functional way to train your obliques. They also train your core to efficiently transfer force from your lower body to upper body. This is because your core plays a large role in rotational strength and power movements like throwing, swinging a golf club, and punching. Chopping-motion exercises efficiently transfer to these movements while working your entire core, especially your internal and external obliques and TVA. The exercises in this chapter will build abs that look good and perform just as well.

1

BODY-WEIGHT OBLIQUE CRUNCH

Level: Foundational

The body-weight oblique crunch takes you back to basics in learning how to target your external obliques with the simplest of movements. The setup position aligns your body and forces to efficiently isolate your obliques. The simplicity of this exercise allows a great connection with your obliques so you can better work them when you add weight or complexity later on.

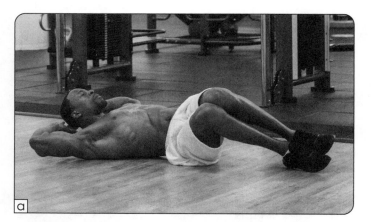

Setup

- Lie on your back on a mat (optional) on the floor.
- Bring your knees together.
- Keep your back as flat on the floor as possible while letting your knees drop to one side.
- Place your hands behind your head or crossed on your chest.

Performance

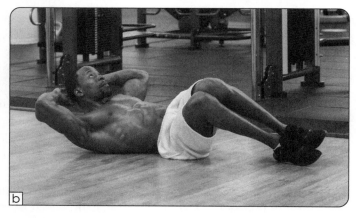

1. Visualize the space between your ribs on one side and your hip on the same side, which is opposite to the side you dropped your knees to.
2. Contract your obliques to pull your ribs to your hip on the same side.
3. Breathe out as you rise into an oblique crunch, exhaling fully as you reach the top.
4. Keep your head neutral throughout.
5. Lower to the start and all the way to the floor.
6. Exhale as you rise and inhale as you lower.
7. Repeat for the desired number of repetitions on each side.

Tips for Success

- To make body-weight oblique crunches even harder, create instability by lifting both of your feet off the floor while your knees remain to one side of your body.
- To place more weight through your midsection, straighten your legs more.

2
SIDE PLANK LIFT

Level: Intermediate

Side plank lifts train your obliques by using a lateral spinal flexion pattern. They also double as an exercise to train your hip abductors, such as your gluteus minimus and medius. They are good for developing chiseled obliques as well as stronger hips and more resilient knees. If you think of these as a basic side plank performed dynamically, you're already most of the way there.

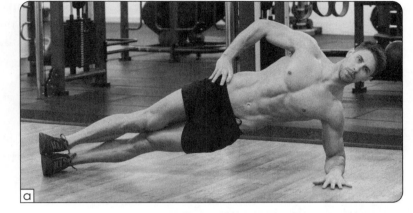

Setup

- Lie on your side with one elbow down and your shoulder aligned directly over it.
- Your body is straight and your feet together.
- Lift your hips and legs off the floor into a basic side plank and hold the position.

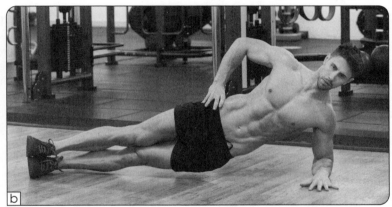

Performance

1. Keeping your feet planted and elbow in place, begin to drop your hip toward the floor.
2. Your hip will hike out somewhat as your spine laterally flexes and your hip adducts (your hip drops bringing your bottom leg in toward the midline of your body).
3. Lower your hip as close to the floor as you can before returning to the starting point, emphasizing hip abduction of your bottom leg and returning back to your body's midline.
4. Repeat the movement, returning each time to the neutral position of the basic side plank.

Tips for Success

- Make side plank lifts more difficult by increasing the range of motion, but only if you are already capable of touching the floor with your bottom hip.
- Raise your planted elbow and feet off the floor by placing them on a small step or a few inches of Olympic plates.
- Perform this exercise with your elbow placed on a regular gym bench.
- To add weight resistance, hold a light plate on the side of your top hip.

3
KNEELING CABLE SIDE CRUNCH

Level: Intermediate

Kneeling crunches are common in many gyms and among people chasing six-pack abs. But kneeling cable side crunches are less common. Adding a small twist to your kneeling crunch emphasizes your obliques because your body position and the cable are better aligned to take your external obliques through to a fully shortened and then lengthened position.

Setup

- Use a V-bar or rope attachment on your cable system.
- Set the cable to approximately chest height when standing.
- Kneel about half your body length away from the cable and to a 30- to 45-degree angle to one side.
- Grab the attachment.

Performance

1. Hold the cable just over the top of your head and keep it there for the duration of the exercise.
2. In your sideways kneeling position, lean in toward the cable, allowing the resistance to hold you up.
3. Crunch down toward one side, closing the space between the cable and your ribs and hip closest to the cable.
4. Do not let your hips sit back when crunching down.
5. Focus on your obliques doing the work and maximally contracting with each rep.
6. Breathe out fully as you reach the bottom position.
7. Come all the way out of the side crunch by stretching your obliques, but do not move your hips.
8. Inhale as you come up.

Tips for Success

A common fault during this exercise is to use your arms to pull the cable down rather than contracting your abs. Initiate the movement by first contracting of your abs.

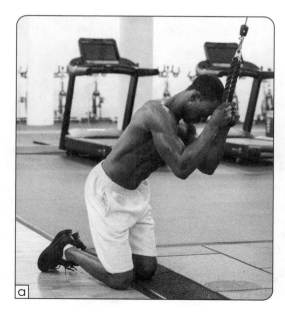
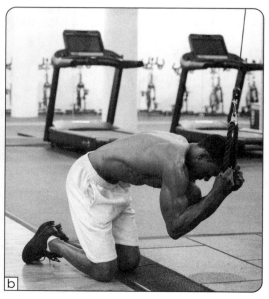

4
BAND ROTATION

Level: Foundational

Band rotations are a foundational exercise and a good way to learn how to correctly perform chopping motions: the efficient transfer of force from your lower body to upper body, ending in a strong and powerful swipe of the resistance band. The proper motion is not simply a rotation of your shoulders. Pay attention to how your knees and hips move in this exercise as your glutes and obliques work together.

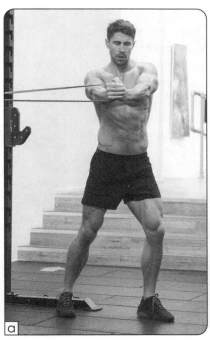 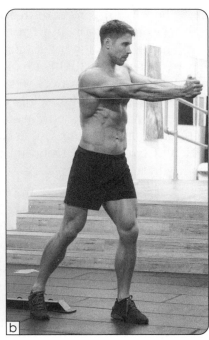

Setup

- Loop a resistance band around something sturdy at shoulder height. A power rack or unused piece of gym equipment is a good option.
- Grab the resistance band with a double-overhand grip and step away from the anchor point.
- The band should be to one side, and your elbows should be straight.
- Place the leg farthest from the anchor point a few feet (about 60 cm) in front of the other leg.
- Stay tall, and engage your core.

Performance

1. Swipe the resistance band horizontally and straight across your body from one side to the other.
2. The back hip (closest to the anchor point) should extend, and if possible, your foot should pivot. Although pivoting your foot is a more advanced option, it is encouraged as good practice.
3. Rotate your spine and shoulders to swipe the band across.
4. Keep your core braced throughout, and focus on making your obliques perform as much of the movement as possible.

Tips for Success

- To make the exercise easier, step closer to the anchor point of the band to decrease the resistance.
- Performing the exercise with more bend in the elbows allows you to use a heavier band or makes a lighter band feel easier.
- Don't forget to breathe! The high tension created through your hips and core can make this exercise a challenge if you aren't breathing with each repetition.

5
CABLE CHOP

Level: Intermediate

Cable chops train your core in a rotational movement pattern, working your internal and external obliques as well as the TVA and other muscles around the hips. They're considered a highly functional movement, with excellent transfer to a variety of daily and athletic movements. Taking a deeper look into cable chops, you'll see how they require hip extension on one side and internal hip rotation on the other. Golfers and tennis players in particular can benefit from improving strength and stability in this movement.

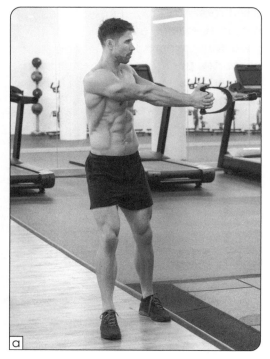

Setup

- Start with a cable set at shoulder height and a single handle attached.
- Grab the handle and step away from it to one side.
- Place one foot in front of the other in a staggered stance and feet approximately shoulder-width apart.
- The back foot should be on the side nearest the cable.
- The arms are straight, with a slight bend at the elbows, not locked.
- Stabilize your hips, knees, and spine by engaging your core and glutes.

Performance

1. Swipe the cable horizontally across your body from one side to the other.
2. Extend the back hip and raise that heel from the floor.
3. Rotate you spine and shoulders as you move the cable from one side to the other.
4. Rotate as far as you can or until the cable just touches your arm.
5. Control the cable back to the start, but do not let the resistance go.
6. Breathe out as you chop across. Breathe in as you return to the start.

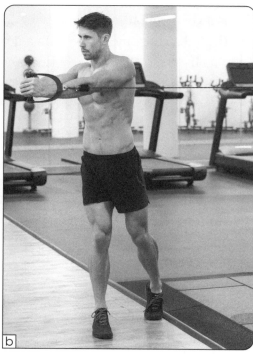

Tips for Success

- Experiment with different stances depending on what you want from the exercise and what feels best.
- Experiment with different cable heights and chopping directions, such as in the cable high chop.

6
CABLE HIGH CHOP

Level: Intermediate

In this exercise, the chop is from a low to high position. The cable handle starts about level with your hips and then finishes overhead. The advantage of performing a cable chop is the emphasis on transferring force from your lower body to upper body. As a builder of obliques, it doesn't hold too much value. But, as a movement with great sport specificity and to develop a more athletic core, this is a good option.

Setup

- Start with a cable set between knee and hip height and a single handle attached.
- Grab the cable with both hands and step away from it to one side.
- Start the cable by your pocket and with arms straight and shoulders back.
- Place one foot in front of the other. Your back foot is on the side of the cable.
- Stabilize your hips, knees, and spine by engaging your core and glutes.

Performance

1. Press your back foot into the floor as you begin to raise the cable from your side to overhead on the opposite side.
2. Start from a low position with bent hips and knees, and move to a reaching position overhead.
3. The action on the way up should be relatively forceful, and the action on the way down should be controlled.
4. Keep your core engaged throughout the exercise.
5. Focus less on feeling the exercise in your obliques and more on exerting force through the floor and the cable.

Tips for Success

For another variation, perform the cable high chop facing toward the cable. The angle and direction of force are useful for martial artists and athletes in sports that involve grappling.

7

BODY-WEIGHT RUSSIAN TWIST

Level: Foundational

The body-weight Russian twist is a foundational exercise similar to a twisting sit-up. The popular Russian twist is typically done with kettlebells or medicine balls or while holding a weight plate. Mastering this exercise with just body weight allows you to perfect your twisting technique so you can feel it in your midsection. After mastering this using just body weight, begin adding weight to the movement while still focusing on feeling it work.

Setup

- Begin lying on a mat (optional) in a basic sit-up position with your feet together.
- Rise to the top of the sit-up position, and place your palms together.
- Your arms should be straight out in front of you.

Performance

1. Rotate your shoulders and arms to one side.
2. Do not let your hips move, and keep your feet facing forward.
3. Your head follows in the direction of your hands to allow your spine to fully rotate to the side.
4. Exhale as you rotate as far you can.
5. Return to the middle before repeating in the opposite direction.
6. Keep your core engaged throughout, and focus on feeling the twisting motion work the obliques.

Tips for Success

Lift your feet off the floor and hover them approximately five inches (13 cm) off the floor for an extra challenge.

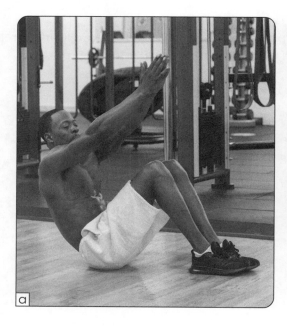
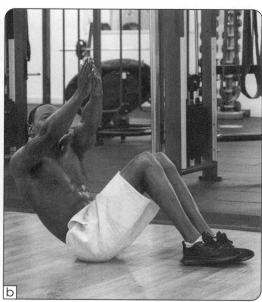

8
KETTLEBELL RUSSIAN TWIST

Level: Intermediate

Once you master the body-weight Russian twist and can feel it through your obliques and entire midsection, add a little weight. A kettlebell is a good place to start. Use the kettlebell Russian twist to work your obliques even harder.

Setup

- Begin lying on a mat (optional) in a basic sit-up position with your feet together.
- Grab a kettlebell by the handles (also known as the *horns*).
- Rise to the top of the sit-up position and press the kettlebell out in front of your body.
- Maintain a slight bend in your elbows throughout the exercise.

Performance

1. Rotate your shoulders and arms to one side with the kettlebell in your hands.
2. Keep your knees pressed firmly together, and do not let your hips move. A trick here is to squeeze something between your thighs, such as a foam pad.
3. Let your head follow in the direction the kettlebell to allow your spine to rotate fully to the side.
4. Exhale fully as you rotate as far as you can.
5. Return to the middle before repeating to the opposite side.

Tips for Success

- To make the exercise more challenging, raise the kettlebell farther above your head as you go from side to side.
- Kettlebell Russian twists may also be done with your feet elevated and together (hardest) or crossed and approximately 5 inches (13 cm) off the floor.

9
LANDMINE RUSSIAN TWIST

Level: Advanced

Using a landmine is a novel way to perform Russian twists. The design of the landmine and its natural path of movement make it perfect for chopping and rotating exercises. The setup of this exercise and the weight of the landmine make this one of the more advanced ways to perform Russian twists.

Setup

- Lock a barbell into a landmine unit on the floor.
- Sit on a mat (optional) positioned under the barbell with your hips level with the end of the bar, and pick it up to your chest.
- Finding the correct position may require trial and error.
- Holding your position at the top of the sit-up, press the landmine away from your body while keeping a slight bend in your elbows.
- Keep your feet and knees together.
- Brace your core.

Performance

1. Rotate your shoulders and the barbell to one side using the natural arcing motion of the landmine.
2. Do not let your hips move, and keep your feet facing forward.
3. The end of the bar will travel from your hip on one side to your hip on the other.
4. Alternate sides without using momentum to move the bar.
5. Breathe the way that feels the most natural for you.

Tips for Success

To challenge yourself, lift your feet off the floor and scissor them in the direction opposite your upper body. As you rotate the landmine to the right, take your feet to the left and vice versa.

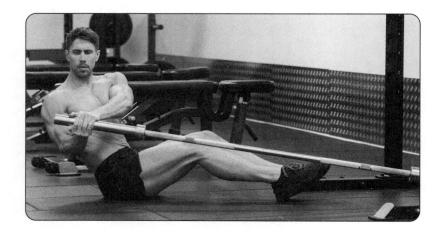

10
INCLINE PLATE RUSSIAN TWIST
Level: Intermediate

Incline plate Russian twists are an intermediate to advanced exercise for your abdominals and obliques. Instead of performing Russian twists flat on the floor, sitting on an incline allows you to maintain abdominal tension for longer. Sitting on a bench can also help you lock in more to target your obliques even harder, and it allows more range of motion when rotating and using a weight plate.

Setup

- Set a bench to a slight incline, and either use a support for your knees or have a partner hold your knees in place.
- Sit on the bench and fix your knees in place according to the type of bench you're using.
- Grab the plate and press it out in front, keeping a slight angle in your elbows.
- Raise one-half to two-thirds of the way up into a sit-up position, and then hold.

Performance

1. Rotate your shoulders and arms to one side with the weight plate in your hands.
2. Your head follows the plate to allow your spine to fully rotate to one side.
3. Return to the middle position, and then repeat on the opposite side.
4. Keep your core engaged throughout, and maintain the same level of rise off the bench.
5. Breathe out on the effort, and breathe in as you lower to the side.

Tips for Success

- The greater the incline, the harder this exercise becomes.
- You can also perform this as a single sit-up into two Russian twists, repeating this each time.

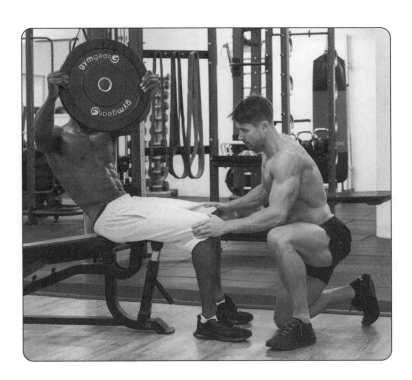

11

STABILITY BALL RUSSIAN TWIST

Level: Intermediate

Stability ball Russian twists require adequate core strength and stability to be able to perform them in a way that benefits your obliques. If you have mastered the simpler Russian twist and have good core awareness, then stability ball Russian twists are an excellent option. They will help build your obliques and core stabilizers at the same time. The stability ball offers comfort and a pivot point to twist over.

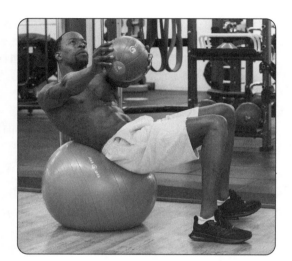

Setup

- Select an appropriately sized stability ball according to manufacturer instructions.
- Sit on top of the stability ball, and hold a lightweight ball or medicine ball.
- Roll yourself down the ball so the middle of your back is resting on it. You may also position the ball farther down in the arch of your lumbar back if that's comfortable.
- Press the weight toward the ceiling with straight arms.
- Position your knees and feet wide to increase support.

Performance

1. Begin to rotate to one side, and allow the ball to roll under you.
2. The ball will roll down the center of your spine toward one side.
3. Rotate your shoulders and spine to one side, taking the weight with you.
4. Don't lose the ball from under you or lose stability.
5. Use your core and obliques to twist back to the starting point with your arms vertical and toward the ceiling again.
6. Keep your core and glutes engaged throughout and your feet firmly locked in place.

Tips for Success

- For more of a locked-in and stable feeling, have a partner hold your knees in place.
- You can also press your knees against a wall to increase stability.
- Performing this exercise on a BOSU ball is a more stable option.

12
HANGING OBLIQUE RAISE

Level: Advanced

Although hanging oblique raises have a relatively low level of complexity, they are an advanced exercise because of the strength required to perform them most effectively. With any hanging leg raise variation, the most important portion of the movement is at the top of the movement. Many athletes don't have enough strength to master that portion of the movement. For this reason, many people swing and use momentum to get to the top of a leg raise instead of engaging the abdominals to do the lifting. Hanging oblique raises are the same. If you have the abdominal and grip strength to perform these correctly, then they're an unbeatable exercise for chiseling your obliques.

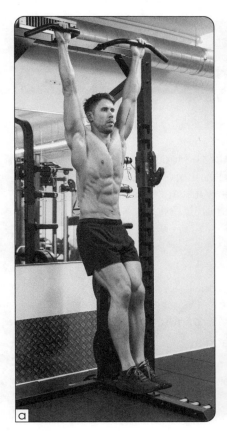
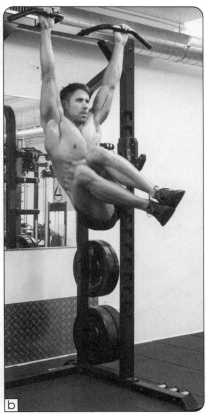

Setup

- Jump up to a bar and hang off it using a double-overhand grip.
- The width of grip can be whatever feels most comfortable for you.
- Keep your shoulders away from your ears by engaging your back.
- Your legs should be straight to begin the exercise.
- Brace your core.

Performance

1. Contract your obliques and begin to raise your knees toward your chest.
2. As you start to bend your knees, begin to turn them to one side.
3. Continue to raise your knees up and toward one side. Instead of pointing forward, your knees should now face slightly more toward one side.
4. Imagine pulling the bar down to engage your lats and help lift your knees.
5. Use your obliques by imagining a pull of your hip toward your ribs on the same side.
6. Raise your knees as high as you can before lowering.
7. Straighten your legs at the bottom, but try to keep them slightly in front.
8. Repeat on the other side.

Tips for Success

- You can make hanging oblique raises more difficult by straightening the legs at the top of the rise.
- You may also use small ankle weights to add progression to the exercise.
- If your lack of grip strength gets in the way of working your abdominals, use wrist wraps or some form of grip assist. As a further progression, try barbell hanging oblique raises.

13
BARBELL HANGING OBLIQUE RAISE

Level: Advanced

Barbell hanging oblique raises take the focus away from your grip and onto your obliques. With more stability and less chance of swinging, there are many advantages to doing this exercise to build chiseled abs and obliques.

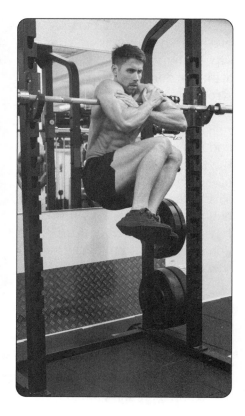

Setup

- Use a Smith machine or a barbell set in a power rack just above shoulder height.
- Place foam pads or a thick towel on the bar for comfort. Do not do this exercise without padding.
- Hook your arms over the padded bar so it is resting in your underarms.
- Place your hands on the opposite shoulders.
- Raise your feet off the floor.

Performance

1. Contract your obliques and begin to raise your knees toward your chest.
2. As you first start bending your knees, begin to turn them toward one side, aiming at the elbow on the opposite side.
3. Continue to raise your knees up and toward one side, ideally all the way to the top to touch an elbow.
4. Use your obliques by imagining a pull of your hip toward your ribs on the same side.
5. Lower to fully straighten your legs, but do not touch the floor.
6. Alternate sides.

Tips for Success

Place a bench in front, lifting your feet over it side to side. This ensures you're getting a good range of motion every time and it adds fun.

14
DUMBBELL SIDE BEND

Level: Intermediate

Dumbbell side bends can be your best friend or your worst enemy. In chapter 2, we discussed how repeated flexions of your spine aren't inherently bad, but anytime you do flex (forward or laterally), you want to ensure you get something out of it. Dumbbell side bends are commonly performed incorrectly, meaning the risks outweigh the benefits. Here's how to make sure you do them in a way that builds your obliques and limits wear and tear.

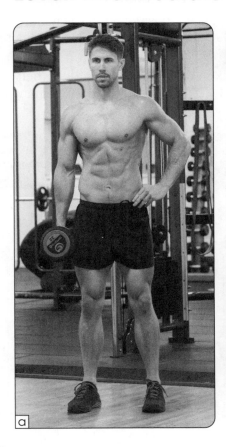 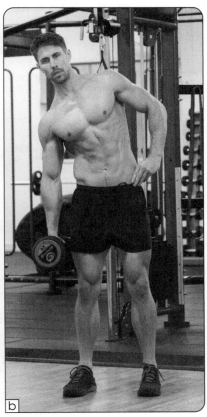

Setup

- Begin in a standing position with your feet shoulder-width apart and a dumbbell in one hand.
- Stand fully upright and do not allow the dumbbell to pull you to one side.
- Brace your core and squeeze your glutes by imagining "spreading the floor" with your feet.

Performance

1. While trying to move within a single plane, begin to bend sideways in the direction of the dumbbell.
2. Allow the dumbbell to pull you down, but work hard to fight any jerking or twisting motion.
3. Take a full two seconds to lower the dumbbell.
4. Lower until you feel a slight stretch in your obliques on the side opposite the dumbbell.
5. Do not lower any farther than you need to, and try to isolate a lateral flexion of your spine only. The range of motion might be less than you think it should be.
6. Contract your obliques on the side without the dumbbell to pull yourself back to the start.
7. The start and finish position is where your torso is fully upright.
8. You do not need to continue your bend in the opposite direction once you start to feel a slight stretch in your obliques.

Tips for Success

- A common flaw with the dumbbell side bend exercise is using two dumbbells. This is a waste of time because the dumbbells apply an equal force against each other, and the weight does very little to load your obliques.

- Another common flaw is bending too far in the direction opposite the dumbbell. Again, this is useless because the dumbbell is not positioned in a way that will load lateral flexion when you travel past upright and in the opposite direction (the load is too close to your spine meaning less torque and reduced muscle tension).

- If you choose to laterally flex in the opposite direction, then a cable is a better option. This is because of the direction of the resistance and a change in moment arm length.

15
TATE SIDE BEND

Level: Intermediate

Side bends with dumbbells and cables are a common lateral flexion movement used to train your obliques. A less common way to train your obliques using a similar movement pattern is to push the weight down instead of pulling it up. One example of this is the Tate side bend, which requires you to press the cable down as you laterally flex your spine. You can use considerable weight with this exercise to effectively target your obliques.

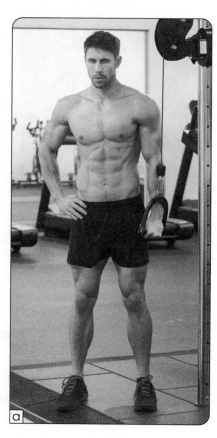
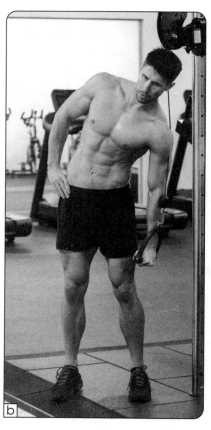

Setup

- Use a height-adjustable cable so the handle can start and finish as close to your torso as possible.

- Set the cable high and attach a single handle.

- Pull the handle down to hip level, keeping your arm straight and fixed by your side.

- Stand with your side toward the cable and your feet comfortably about shoulder-width apart.

- Brace your core, and stay strong in this start–finish position.

Performance

1. Keeping the cable close to the outside of your thigh, press it down by your side using your obliques.
2. Focus on laterally flexing your spine.
3. Squeeze your obliques hard on the way down, and then stretch a little as you rise back to the top.
4. Do not laterally flex in the opposite direction.

Tips for Success

Isolating lateral flexion is the key. A good way to think about laterally flexing your spine is to imagine you're trying to bend sideways, sandwiched between two panes of glass. If you bend forward too much (bend your spine forward or flex your hips), then you headbutt the glass.

16

LOW-CABLE SIDE BEND

Level: Intermediate

The low-cable side bend is an intermediate exercise that works your obliques through a lateral flexion pattern. The goal of these is to isolate lateral flexion and perform side bends without excessive spinal movement or loading.

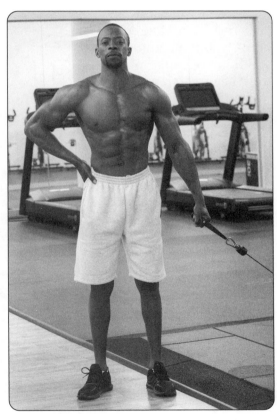

Setup

- Set a cable to a low position and attach a single handle.
- Begin facing sideways to the cable.
- Your feet should be shoulder-width apart, and the cable should be in your nearside hand.
- Stand fully upright, and do not allow the cable to pull you to one side.
- Brace your core and squeeze your glutes by imagining "spreading the floor" with your feet.

Performance

1. While trying to move in a single plane, begin to bend sideways in the direction of the cable.
2. Allow the cable to pull you down, but do so under control.
3. Bend down until you feel a slight stretch in your obliques on the side opposite the cable.
4. The range of motion will likely be less than you think it should be.
5. Contract your obliques on the noncable side to pull yourself back to the upright starting position.
6. You may continue to bend in the opposite direction very slightly. This is optional and depends on whether it feels good for you.

Tips for Success

- Changing the height of the cable can change the point of maximal loading.
- Using a low cable will work you hardest in a more bent-over position (greater degree of lateral flexion and lengthened obliques).
- Setting the cable gradually higher will work you hardest in a more upright position (lesser degree of lateral flexion and shortened obliques).
- Use cable side bend variations to work your obliques harder or easier at different muscle lengths.

17
KETTLEBELL WINDMILL

Level: Advanced

Kettlebell windmills are popular among kettlebell training enthusiasts and for good reason. They work to open out your hips and posterior chain while developing shoulder and core stability. Because of the way they stretch and load your obliques, they are a useful exercise for building them up, too. Kettlebell windmills are a good all-around exercise, but their complexity when done correctly gives them status as an advanced exercise.

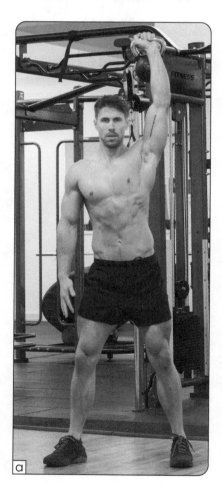
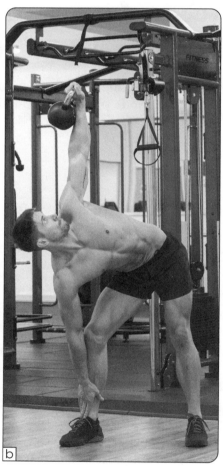

Setup

- Grip a kettlebell in one hand and press it overhead.
- Your feet are just wider than shoulder-width apart. Adjust this depending on what feels best.
- Slightly turn out the foot on the opposite side of the kettlebell.
- Keep your eyes on the kettlebell at all times.

Performance

1. Initiate the movement by pushing back your hip on the side of the kettlebell and slightly to the side.
2. Your free hand is on the inside of your turned-out leg.

3. As you push your hip back, your hand traces down the inside of the opposite leg and toward the floor.

4. Bow over while keeping your spine neutral and knees at the same angle.

5. Keep the kettlebell pressed overhead. As you come down, your arm stays vertical, strongly holding the kettlebell overhead.

6. Lower as far as you can without bending your knees or spine. You should feel a stretch on one side of your body.

7. Return to the top with an exhale.

8. You can practice without a kettlebell to start with.

Tips for Success

- You can use kettlebell windmills as a warm-up exercise to open out your hips and backside before lower-body and core-focused workouts. For more on how to structure your warm-ups refer to chapter 12.

- You may also perform this exercise with a dumbbell.

18
HALF-KNEELING DUMBBELL WINDMILL

Level: Advanced

The half-kneeling dumbbell windmill is an advanced core exercise that requires coordination and stability. It's also an effective exercise for loading and stretching your obliques at the same time. If you want to limit lateral flexion and still work your obliques hard, then windmill variations are useful. Performing from a half-kneeling rather than a standing position manages restrictions you might have in your flexibility. Half-kneeling windmills are also self-limiting because you must touch the floor each time for successful completion of each repetition.

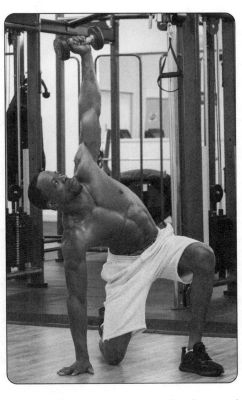

Setup

- Adopt a half-kneeling position on the floor.
- Grip a dumbbell in the hand of the forward leg and press it overhead.
- The opposite hand rests in front of your back thigh.
- Keep your eyes on the dumbbell at all times.

Performance

1. Maintain the 90-degree angle in your front and back knees throughout.

2. Hinge your hips to bend your torso over, allowing your free hand to travel down the front of your back thigh.

3. Press the dumbbell firmly overhead with your arm perpendicular to the floor as you lower all the way down.

4. Bend over as far as you can or until you can touch the floor with your free hand.
5. You should feel a stretch in your hips and obliques.
6. Return to the start by raising your torso.
7. Keep your knuckles pointing toward the ceiling.
8. Exhale as you rise.

Tips for Success

If achieving this range of motion is difficult, then place a foam pad or yoga block in front of your back thigh. You can stop lowering when your free hand touches the pad or block. Try to get deeper over time to work your obliques even harder at the bottom.

19
SUSPENDED OBLIQUE TUCK

Level: Intermediate

Suspended oblique tucks are a knee tuck with a twist. Literally. Set up in your regular knee tuck position using a suspension trainer and then pull your knees in toward your chest with a slight twisting motion. This causes your obliques to work that much harder as you extend your hips on the way back, creating a useful antiextension core exercise.

Setup

- Set a suspension trainer 6 to 10 inches (15-25 cm) from the floor.
- Get into a basic push-up position and place your feet into the stirrups of the suspension trainer.
- Your head, shoulders, and hips should be level, and your core should be braced.

Performance

1. Begin by tucking your knees up toward your chest and to one side.
2. Imagine bringing your knees up and toward your opposite elbow in a slight twisting motion.
3. Your pelvis will tuck somewhat as you bring your knees farther up. This is encouraged.
4. Exhale as you pull your knees in before returning to the starting position.

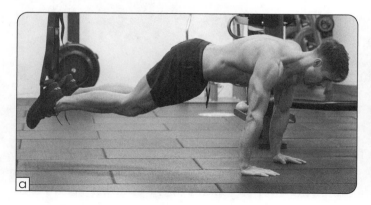
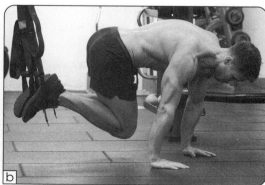

Tips for Success

- The farther you walk your hands from the suspension trainer anchor point, the harder the exercise becomes.
- For a novel and even more challenging variation, try this exercise using thick resistance bands instead of a suspension trainer.

20
SIDE-TO-SIDE MEDICINE BALL SLAM

Level: Intermediate

Side-to-side medicine ball slams are an intermediate-level exercise that incorporates explosiveness into your ab and core workouts. They won't carve out your obliques as much as other exercises will, but instead they will help you build explosive power and athleticism. Other exercises will build the *show*, while slam variations will give you the *go*.

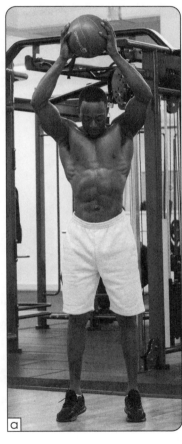
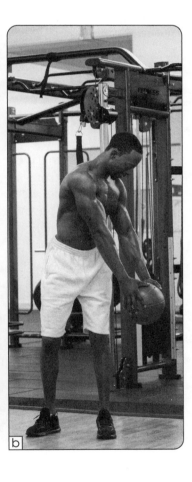

Setup

- Stand with a heavy medicine ball in your hands. For most people, five to eight kilograms is a good starting point.
- Your feet should be about shoulder-width apart.

Performance

1. Raise the medicine ball overhead with both hands and allow your heels to leave the floor; think "get big."
2. Pull the ball down as hard and fast as you can toward one side of your body.
3. Aim the ball just outside and in front of your foot. This naturally becomes a slight lateral flexion and rotation movement.
4. Think "Drive the ball through the floor."
5. Let the ball bounce before catching it.
6. Arc the ball over your head and repeat immediately on the other side in a side-to-side motion.

Tips for Success

A heavier ball is not always better. Pick a weight that allows you to maintain the same speed from the first to the last repetition. The goal is maximal power, not fatigue and messy-looking slams.

21
MEDICINE BALL ROTATIONAL TOSS

Level: Intermediate

The medicine ball rotational toss is a power-based chopping exercise. It teaches efficient transfer of force from your hip through your core and finishes with a medicine ball firing off into the wall. Use this exercise to mix up your core workouts, for transfer to athletic movements, or just to take out some aggression on a wall!

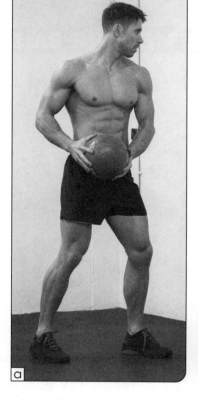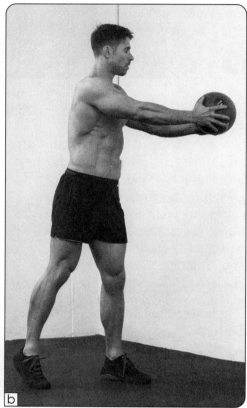

Setup

- Begin three to five feet (1-1.5 m) from a wall. Adjust the distance depending on the bounce of the ball and your catching ability.
- Stand in a staggered stance with one foot in front of the other approximately shoulder-width apart and with a slight bend in both knees.
- Hold a medicine ball with both hands close to your back hip.
- A three- to five-kilogram medicine ball is a good starting point.

Performance

1. In an explosive rotational movement, throw the ball as hard as you can from your back hip to the wall.
2. Your hips will punch through as your spine and shoulders rotate.
3. When the ball is released, keep your hands in front of you, ready to catch it again.
4. Catch the ball and return it back to the same side hip.
5. Immediately repeat on the same side, allowing as little time as possible between repetitions.
6. The absorption and release of the ball between each repetition should be like a spring.

Tips for Success

- You can also perform this exercise alternating sides and requiring a fast transition of your stance between repetitions.
- Try low-to-high ball tosses or ball tosses directly facing the wall for variation.

22
LANDMINE HALF-CORE-ROTATION

Level: Advanced

Landmines are ideally suited to rotational and chopping actions because of their unique design. Start the landmine half-core-rotation exercise in a typical chopping position much like you'd perform with cables. But the landmine uses a low-to-high chopping motion that requires tremendous hip and core strength. The half-core-rotation exercise finishes in the middle before lowering, whereas the landmine full-core-rotation (the next exercise) is more complex. Both are considered advanced exercises.

Setup

- Place a barbell in a landmine unit.
- Pick up the barbell and hold it away from your chest.
- Stand in a staggered stance with one foot in front of the other approximately shoulder-width apart.
- Keep your chest proud and eyes focused on the end of the barbell.
- Brace your core throughout.

Performance

1. Lower the barbell into an arcing motion and toward your back hip.
2. Keep your arms straight as your shoulders and spine rotate.
3. Allow your hips to absorb the weight as you reach the bottom position. Keep your shoulders back and your chest proud.
4. Reverse the motion by rotating the barbell and landmine unit back to the start position.
5. Rotate your shoulders and spine as your hips extend to lift the bar.

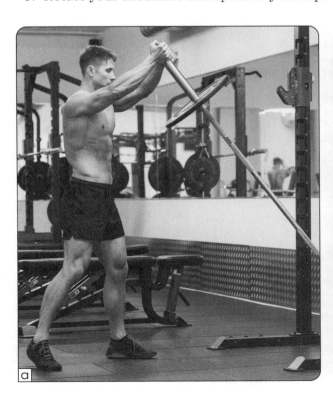
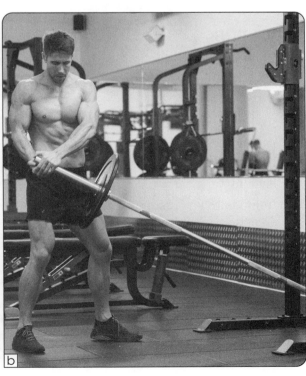

6. The heel of your back leg may leave the floor in the final part of the lift. This is optional, but recommended.

7. Breathe in as you lower, and then breathe out as you forcefully lift the bar back to the middle.

Tips for Success

Perform the landmine half-core-rotation exercise with one knee on the floor in a half-kneeling position. This requires greater core and rotational strength because it's mechanically harder to move the landmine from this position. The half-kneeling position also stops your legs and hips from helping as much.

23
LANDMINE FULL-CORE-ROTATION

Level: Advanced

The landmine full-core-rotation exercise is fun and effective if you get it right. This exercise is advanced for a reason: It requires good core strength and full-body coordination to rotate the landmine efficiently and switch it from one side to the other. Compare this is to the half-core-rotation exercise, which works only one side at a time and does not require a full rotation of the barbell. For solid obliques and full-body athleticism, the landmine full-core-rotation is hard to beat.

Setup

- Place a barbell in a landmine unit.
- Pick up the barbell and hold it away from your chest.
- Stand with your feet wider than shoulder width and with slightly bent knees. Face the landmine unit.
- Keep your chest proud and eyes focused on the end of the barbell.
- Brace your core throughout.

Performance

1. Lower the barbell into an arcing motion and toward your hip on one side.
2. Keep your arms straight as your shoulders and spine rotate toward that side.
3. Allow your hips to absorb the weight as the end of the bar moves closer toward your thigh.
4. As you do this, take a slight step back on that same side to better absorb the weight.
5. Do not let your spine flex forward, and keep your chest up and proud throughout.
6. Reverse the motion by rotating the barbell and landmine unit back to the middle, moving your back foot forward to its original position.
7. Immediately transition onto the other side, allowing the barbell to continue its travel in that direction.
8. Switch your body position to mirror what was done on the other side.

Tips for Success

At its core, this exercise is simply a left-to-right chop with the landmine. Do not overthink it. If you have built the required foundation and coordination, then the movement should come naturally. If you haven't, then you're in for a challenge.

24
HIGH-CABLE SIDE BEND

Level: Intermediate

The action of the high-cable side bend is similar to that of a dumbbell or low-cable side bend. The main difference is in the position of the cable held behind your head. This changes the point of maximal load so the movement is most challenging when you're closer to an upright position (the top). Compare this to a low-cable side bend or a dumbbell side bend, where the side bend is most challenging the more you flex over to one side (the bottom). Training muscles at different joint angles and lengths is an important consideration when trying to build strong muscles and a more resilient body.

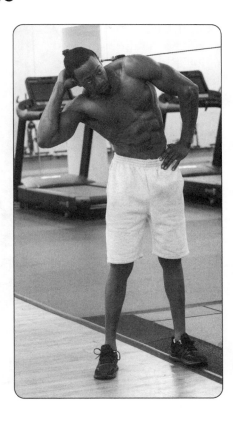

Setup

- Set a cable to forehead height and attach a single handle.
- Begin standing sideways to the cable with your feet shoulder-width apart.
- Hold the cable in the hand farthest from the cable stack and behind your head. It will remain there for the duration of the exercise.
- You should be fully upright, and don't allow the cable to pull you toward it.
- Brace your core and squeeze your glutes by "spreading the floor" with your feet.

Performance

1. Begin to bend sideways in the direction away from the cable.
2. Laterally flex your spine as far as you can and to whatever degree is comfortable.
3. The range of motion will likely be less than you think it should be.
4. Contract your obliques as you laterally flex.
5. Return to the fully upright position, controlling the cable on the way back.

Tips for Success

High-cable side bends also work well with a resistance band instead of a cable.

25
HEAVY BATTLE ROPE STRIKE

Level: Intermediate

Battle ropes are largely used as a conditioning and calorie-burning tool. But heavy battle ropes can also be considered another way to apply resistance to your body. Heavier, longer, or thicker ropes offer a form of progressive overload just like picking up a heavier weight. And the heavier the battle rope, the slower the movement and the more force you have to apply. Rather than speed, this exercise is about brute strength and explosiveness. Heavy battle rope strikes use a powerful chopping action that will add variety and athleticism to your full-body and oblique-focused workouts.

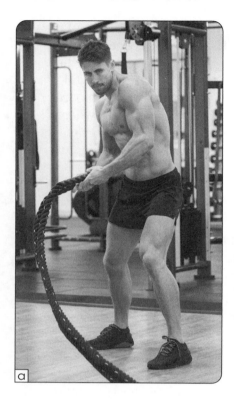
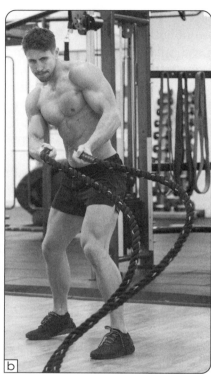

Setup

- Grab the end of both battle ropes with a palms-down grip. You'll be working one side of your body at a time.
- Place one foot in front of the other, angling yourself approximately 45 degrees to the rope anchor.
- The feet are six inches (15 cm) apart from each other and parallel.

Performance

1. Strike both ropes with both hands horizontally in a movement that looks somewhat like a backhand in tennis.
2. Allow your back hip to punch through as your spine and shoulders rotate to whip the ropes.
3. If performed correctly, you'll produce sideways waves in both of the ropes at the same time.
4. Repeat this explosive action on one side and without a break between repetitions.

Tips for Success

- Use different angles on your battle rope strikes to mix up your training and muscle emphasis.
- Low-to-high and high-to-low strikes are good options.

26
HEAVY BATTLE ROPE UPPERCUT

Level: Intermediate

Heavy battle rope uppercuts build a powerful core and hips while allowing you to bring out your inner Rocky Balboa. These also work well as part of your conditioning and calorie-burning workouts (see chapter 4).

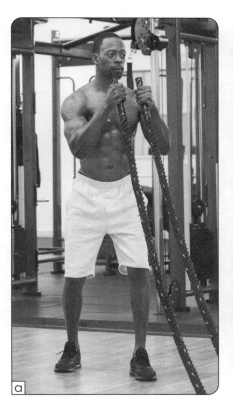
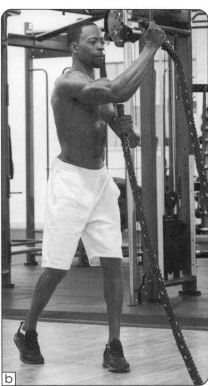

Setup

- Hold the battle ropes in both hands using a thumbs-up grip.
- Stand in a staggered stance with one foot in front of the other approximately shoulder-width apart.
- Slightly bend your hips and knees, but keep your shoulders back and chest proud.

Performance

1. With the hand positioned on the back leg only, punch the rope up into an uppercut. This will be a low-to-high chop of one arm and with the palm of your hand facing toward you.
2. Your back hip will punch through as your knees and hips extend and finish with a powerful punch of your arm.
3. Repeat all of your repetitions on one side before immediately switching to the other.

Tips for Success

- Heavy battle rope uppercuts can also be done with alternating arms. This requires coordination so the ropes don't hit each other.
- For conditioning and calorie-burning workouts, use lighter ropes and shorten your rest periods.
- To build brute force and a battle-ready core, "Go hard or go home!"

Chapter 10

Planks and Other "Anti" Movements

In chapter 3, we identified the clear difference between core training and ab training. To summarize, your core is made up of many muscles that stabilize and control movement around your spine, pelvis, and hips. Your abdominals, although part of your core, contribute much less to performance and more to aesthetics.

A chiseled midsection is created by working the abdominals specifically and is made visible by also having a low percentage of body fat. On the other hand, an athlete's ability to handle large forces or a race car driver's resilience against spine-bending g-forces requires great core strength. While this book focuses on how to attain an impressive-looking midsection, for best results in the long run, you should also train your core as a whole unit. This will ensure that your six-pack abs are part of a strong and healthy core.

To improve your core strength, you must develop spinal stability in all directions. Planks are just one example of a core exercise, and you'll learn that they train you in just one direction and position—a position that has limited real-world application. Variations of these exercises, though, as well as others covered in this section will show you how to train in the most efficient way to enhance core strength and spinal stability in all directions.

The majority of exercises in this chapter emphasize maintaining good spinal and pelvic alignment. Your focus should be on keeping your spine stable while limiting excessive movement in any direction. Optimal setup and performance is described in each exercise, and photos also help to identify what ideal positioning looks like during these exercises.

Some exercises also require different breathing patterns, or a reminder to ensure you are breathing in the first place. For these exercises, the ideal breathing pattern is described. However, overall any breathing is better than no breathing at all. So, in most cases, you should breathe with whatever pattern is most comfortable for you.

Because of the nature of core exercises and their role in developing spinal stability, these exercises are often referred to as "anti" movements. We can use the following categories to classify your core exercises according to which movement you're resisting. Performing exercises from all the categories will improve your overall programming and make sure you leave no stone (or movement direction) unturned:

- *Antirotation:* In these exercises, your core resists the rotation of your spine, pelvis, and hips. Examples are the cable Pallof press (page 195 and eccentric one-arm push-up (page 180).

- *Anti-lateral-flexion:* In these exercises, your core resists the lateral flexion of your spine and a sideways drop of your hip (lateral pelvic tilt). Examples are the basic side plank (page 162) and one-arm farmer's carry (page 165).

- *Antiextension:* These exercises engage your core in order to resist spinal extension and a forward tilt of your pelvis (anterior pelvic tilt). Examples include the slider body saw (page 177) and dead-stop ab wheel rollout (page 170).

- *Antiflexion:* Often a forgotten component within core training, antiflexion exercises train your core to resist spinal flexion and posterior pelvic tilt. Examples are found in chapter 11 in the complementary exercises section.

While we can classify core exercises using these categories, it is important to note that most effective core exercises don't fit into just one category. You can classify an exercise according to the main movement it resists, but it will likely cross over into another category as well. For example, when performing a plank and lifting one leg into the air, you are developing antiextension strength, but the leg lift adds an antirotational component to the exercise. In most cases, this is a positive as far as training efficiency goes and will help you hit multiple categories at the same time. Consider these categories in your core training plans and ensure you cover all of your bases. This does not always require a long list of exercises, just a few of the most efficient ones.

1
BASIC FRONT PLANK

Level: Foundational

The basic front plank is a foundational core exercise used mostly to develop the endurance of your spinal stabilizers in an antiextension capacity. Basic front planks are a poor choice for aesthetic purposes, and their specificity to real-world activities is limited. However, the endurance of your deep spinal stabilizers is important for spinal health and maintaining upright posture. For that reason, the basic front plank is a useful exercise for beginners. Basic front planks also transfer to other exercises done in the same plane. For example, push-ups benefit when you can perform a front plank correctly.

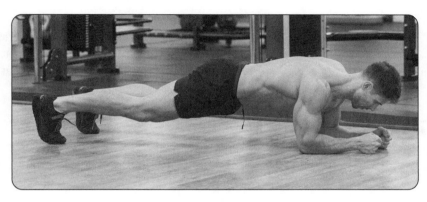

Setup

- Lie facedown on the floor.
- Place your elbows on the ground about shoulder-width apart and push yourself up to stack your shoulders directly over your elbows.
- Clench your fists.
- Keep your knees and hips down as you place your feet about hip-width apart. The closer together your feet, the more unstable your basic front plank will be.

Performance

1. Assume the full front-plank position with your toes pressed into the floor and knees and hips lifted.
2. Support your weight on your elbows and toes.
3. Your entire spine is neutral and level between your head, shoulders, spine, and hips.
4. Brace your core; imagine 360 degrees of air around your spine and contracted abs.
5. Pinch your glutes together to help keep your hips fully extended.
6. Hold this position and control your breathing throughout the hold.

Tips for Success

- Holding a basic front plank for a long time, while impressive, will do little for your physique or performance.
- Holding planks for longer than one minute increases muscular endurance.
- Use holds of up to 40 seconds, and don't be afraid to add resistance if this is too easy.
- Setting a weight comfortably across your hips is the best way to add load to your basic front plank. This load should be spread evenly between your hips and lower back.

2
LONG-LEVER PLANK

Level: Advanced

The long-lever plank is a more advanced version of the basic front plank, which offers some people little challenge. The increase in difficulty is made possible by an increase in lever length. The elbows and feet are farther from each other and the position is narrower. This requires your core to work much harder to resist spinal extension and anterior pelvic tilt. Other nuances of this exercise add to its difficulty as well.

Setup

- Lie facedown on the floor.
- Place your elbows together on the floor; ideally, they are touching.
- Keep your knees on the floor for now, but position your feet so they are touching.

Performance

1. Push through your toes and elbows to move into a plank position.
2. Clench your glutes and abs hard.
3. Walk your elbows forward until they are under your forehead, and make sure they are still together. This position creates a plank with a longer lever.
4. Clench your fists hard and imagine pulling your elbows toward your toes and toes toward your elbows. This engages your lats and abdominals further.
5. Keep your glutes pinched together and core braced.
6. Shaking at this point is not uncommon.
7. Hold this position and maintain alignment between your shoulders, back, spine, and hips.
8. Do not let your lower back sag into extension or hips to drop too low.

Tips for Success

Clenching your fists hard and squeezing your shoulder blades together on any plank variation instantly makes it harder without requiring extra equipment.

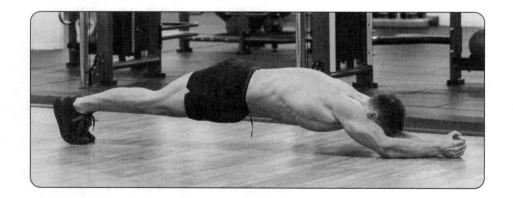

3
STIR THE POT

Level: Intermediate

The stir the pot exercise is a basic front plank with a dynamic component added. Your elbows are placed on a stability ball and move in a lateral figure-8 motion. As your elbow position shifts, your core works to resist rotation and the tilt of your pelvis and spine. The wider your elbows travel and higher they go, the more the demand increases. Exercises like these are transferable to daily activities because your core has to stabilize your spine and pelvis in the presence of a changing environment.

Setup

- Select an appropriately sized stability ball according to manufacturer instructions.
- Start by kneeling in front of the stability ball with your elbows on the middle and slightly narrower than shoulder-width apart.

Performance

1. Push your toes into the floor and your hips up as you press your elbows into the ball.
2. Your hips should be up and your body in a solid plank position.
3. Hold here and stabilize for just a second, ensuring you have full control of your body and ball before you start.
4. Keep your glutes pinched together and core braced.
5. Your shoulders, back, spine, and hips should be aligned.
6. Begin to draw a sideways figure-8 with your elbows. This is the stir-the-pot action that will cause the stability ball to move.
7. As your elbows and the ball move, your job is to maintain a relatively static spine and pelvis. In essence, your elbows move, but the rest of your body remains still.
8. Be sure to breathe throughout.

Tips for Success

Instead of using a stability ball, you can also perform the stir-the-pot exercise using a suspension trainer. This is a more advanced variation.

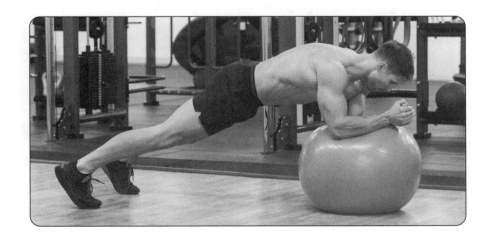

4
MIYAGI PLANK

Level: Intermediate

In the words of karate master Mr. Miyagi from the *Karate Kid* movie, "Wax on, wax off!" Miyagi planks are an intermediate exercise performed using core sliders. The circular motion of "waxing" the floor with each hand adds a dynamic core stabilization component. As well as being an effective antiextension and antirotation exercise, added novelty makes it fun and appealing to perform.

Setup

- Start by kneeling on the floor with both hands placed in front of you on a pair of core sliders.
- The core sliders should be on a surface that allows them to slide.
- If you don't have access to core sliders, use paper plates or put socks over your hands.

Performance

1. Push your toes into the floor and lift your knees to adopt a basic front plank.
2. Place your feet hip-width apart.
3. Position your hands about shoulder-width apart. Your wrists, elbows, and shoulders should be aligned over them.
4. Brace your core and pinch your glutes together to maintain a stable spine and alignment between your hips, back, and neck.
5. Begin to draw a small circle on the floor with one slider, followed by the other in a "wax on, wax off" motion. Your left hand will draw a counterclockwise circle, while your right hand will draw a clockwise circle.
6. Maintain stability in the spine and hips as your arms move.

Tips for Success

- Miyagi planks can also be adjusted for beginners by performing them from the knees.
- To make Miyagi planks more difficult, place a load over your hips.

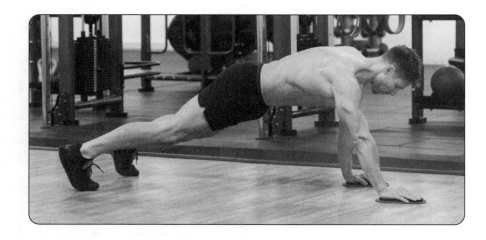

5
SLIDER PLANK WALK

Level: Intermediate

Slider plank walks might look a little different from your more conventional core exercises, but they'll fire up your entire core and give your lungs a great workout at the same time. The aim of this exercise is to maintain a solid plank position and stable pelvis and spine while your hands do the walking and your feet slide along the floor. Moving your hands adds an antirotational component to the plank, while the friction of the floor increases the challenge to resist spinal extension. You'll need adequate space for this one, but it's sure to become your favorite plank variation.

Setup

- Start by kneeling on the floor with both feet placed on a pair of core sliders.
- The core sliders should be on a surface that enables them to slide.
- Make sure you have enough space in front of you to travel at least 10 feet (3 m).

Performance

1. Get into a basic front plank and place your feet on the sliders.
2. Position your hands shoulder-width apart and your feet about hip-width apart.
3. Maintain head, spine, and hip alignment throughout.
4. Begin to walk your hands forward, allowing your feet and the sliders to travel along the floor.
5. Resist the twist of your hips and spine as you travel.
6. Travel forward at least 10 feet (3 m) before reversing the motion.
7. Press your hands into the floor to move in the opposite direction. Keep the front-plank position strong and stable throughout.

Tips for Success

- These are best done for a set amount of time rather than a certain number of repetitions; 10 feet is the minimum space required, but ideally you would use more.
- For a more advanced variation, do the exercise with one foot on a core slider and the other one in the air. This increases the antirotational component and significantly challenges your overall core strength and stability.

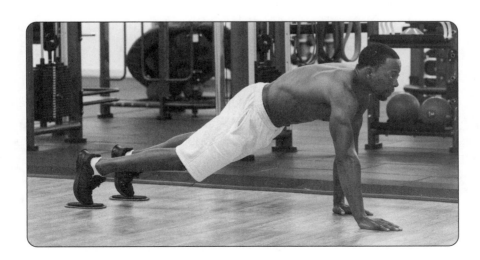

6
BASIC SIDE PLANK

Level: Foundational

The basic side plank is first and foremost an anti-lateral-flexion (spine) exercise that also engages your hip abductors, such as your gluteals. Being strong in exercises that move forward and backward (sagittal plane) is important. But sideways (frontal plane) movements are also important and are more often than not neglected in training plans.

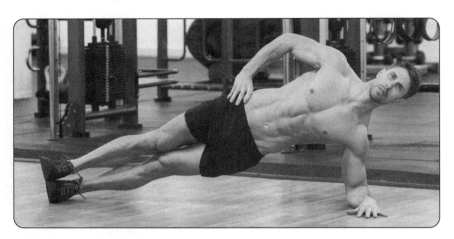

As a frontal plane movement, the basic side plank has an advantage over the basic front plank in that it develops core strength and spinal stability in the sideways direction. As a foundational movement, this exercise helps you develop the prerequisite strength for other core exercises described later in this chapter.

Setup

- Lie on your side on the floor with your elbow down and forearm flat on the floor.
- Stack one foot on top of the other, and position your body in a long straight line.
- You may stagger your feet if you prefer the stability.
- Place your free hand on your hip or by your side.

Performance

1. Take the weight of your body through your planted elbow and feet.
2. Push your hip off the floor to form a sideways bridge.
3. Attempt to create a straight line from your nose, to your belly button, and through the space between your ankles.
4. Looking from above, your head, spine, and hips should be aligned.
5. Brace your core and engage your glutes, lats, and hip abductors to maintain this position.
6. To start, use the breathing technique that feels most comfortable.

Tips for Success

- The basic side plank is a useful way to train in the frontal plane.
- To make this exercise even harder using just your body weight, lift your top leg to create a starlike shape. In this position, your weight is supported only by your bottom leg, which has to work hard to resist hip adduction (hip collapsing toward the floor as your leg travels toward the midline of your body).
- Another way to make the exercise more challenging is to hold a weight on your hip.

7
FACEDOWN CHINESE PLANK

Level: Intermediate

The facedown Chinese plank is a little-known plank variation that trains the ability to resist spinal extension and anterior pelvic tilt. Unlike the basic front plank, it does not require you to support yourself on your arms. This is the main difference and one that allows the performer to focus on stabilizing the hips and

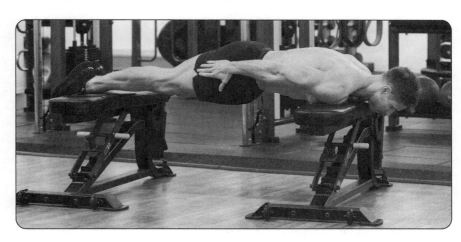

pelvic. If you are more advanced, you will likely find yourself able to handle more weight over your hips when performing the facedown Chinese plank than when performing a weighted front plank. This is because supporting yourself through your chest while facedown on a bench is more stable. Some people find the body position of the facedown Chinese plank to be awkward, while others enjoy achieving the high core tension of this exercise.

Setup

- Place two boxes or benches on the floor approximately a body-length apart.
- Position yourself facedown so your chest rests on one bench and your shins rest on the other.

Performance

1. Create a bridge with your body between the two benches.
2. Your head is off the end of one bench, your feet are off the other, and your arms are straight and close in by your sides.
3. Align your head, back, spine, and hips.
4. Squeeze your glutes and brace your core to maintain the hold.
5. Resist dropping your hips or letting your lower back sag.
6. Press your hands hard into your sides for extra whole-body tension.

Tips for Success

- Increase the difficulty of the facedown Chinese plank by placing weight over your hips.
- When you begin, ask a partner to put a weight plate across your hips.
- Lifting chains are also an excellent loading option because they are comfortable and add instability.
- To make the facedown Chinese plank easier, bring the benches or boxes closer to each other. As you get better over time, move them farther apart.

8

HAND WALKOUT

Level: Intermediate

You may have heard of an abdominal wheel and ab rollouts. If you haven't, then check out the variations later in this chapter. Hand walkouts are the body-weight equivalent of ab wheel rollouts. For that reason, they are easily accessible and require no equipment. And, much like ab wheel rollouts, they achieve high levels of muscle activation throughout your core. Easily scalable for both beginners and advanced athletes, you can walk your hands only part the way or all the way overhead to really fire up your core. Try these to develop your antiextension strength and stability.

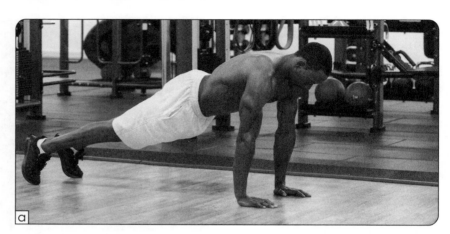

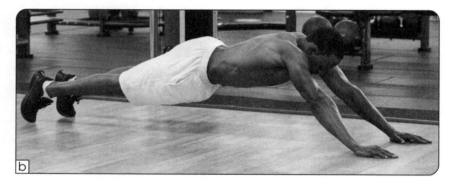

Setup

- Start in the basic front plank position, but on your hands rather than elbows.
- Place your feet shoulder-width apart.
- Align your hips, back, spine, and head.
- Pinch your glutes together, and engage the core.
- Place your hands under your shoulders to begin.

Performance

1. Initiate the movement by walking your hands forward, one hand at a time.
2. Maintain a strong core and stable spine throughout.
3. Walk your hands as far forward as you can. If you feel pain or discomfort, you've gone too far.
4. Walk your hands back to the starting position.
5. One repetition consists of fully walking out then back to the start.

Tips for Success

- Hand walkouts are an ideal body-weight variation for abdominal rollouts using an ab wheel or barbell.
- To make these easier, set up in front of a wall so the wall can act as a stopping point. This means you won't go farther than your core strength can handle.

- Make these harder by holding the bottom position longer or by adding weight. The most efficient way to add weight is to wear a weighted vest.
- You can also perform hand walkouts by finishing in a fully standing position to increase the challenge for your legs.

9
ONE-ARM FARMER'S CARRY

Level: Foundational

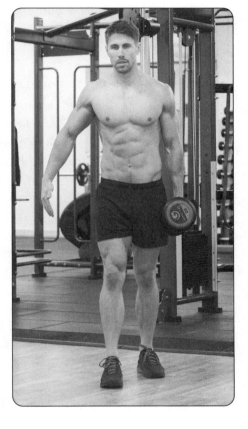

Farmer's carries are a highly functional exercise that have excellent transfer to real-world and sporting activities. They can achieve high levels of overall core muscle activation, including the transverse abdominis, internal and external obliques, and a host of other important spinal stabilizers. Carrying a dumbbell in just one hand adds an anti-lateral-flexion component to the carry, and it requires less weight than you'd otherwise carry using both hands. Learning to resist lateral flexion and hip drop when holding weight on just one side carries over to activities such as holding a grocery bag, carrying a child on one hip, and many sporting movements.

Setup

- Grip a dumbbell in one hand.
- Stand tall, pull your shoulders back, and brace your core.

Performance

1. Go for a walk.
2. Keep a tight grip on the dumbbell, stay tall, and keep your shoulders back.
3. Walk proud and with purpose.
4. Keep your core braced and resist the force of the dumbbell pulling you to one side.
5. Walk forward in a straight line and then back with the dumbbell in the same hand before switching to the other.

Tips for Success

- A good goal to aim for in the one-arm farmer's carry is to carry approximately one-third of your body weight in one hand. If performing a regular farmer's carry with two dumbbells, aim to carry half of your own body weight in each hand.
- Farmer's carries are traditionally done in a straight line, but you can also walk in various directions and patterns—for example, around cones in a figure-8, zigzag, or T-shaped pattern.
- If your space is limited, walk forward and backward in as little as six feet (1.8 m) of space.
- Marching on the spot with the dumbbell in one hand is also a good option when space is limited.

10
HALF-KNEELING BAND ISOMETRIC HOLD

Level: Intermediate

The goal of half-kneeling exercises is to learn how to optimally align your ribs and pelvis so they stack to create a canisterlike effect that engages your core and stabilizes your spine. Many movements can be done from this half-kneeling position. One includes an antirotational component and the use of a resistance band. The half-kneeling band isometric hold develops a bulletproof core and a healthy spine and hips.

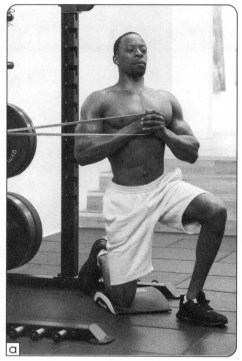

Setup

- Loop a band around a power rack or sturdy upright.
- Use a foam pad or exercise mat on the floor for added comfort for your back knee (optional).
- Get into a half-kneeling position and place your back knee on the foam pad. The back knee is on the side where the band is fixed.
- Both knees are bent approximately 90 degrees; your front foot is flat on the floor and back foot is dorsiflexed (as if it were in starting blocks).
- Bring your torso upright with shoulders back and spine tall.

Performance

1. Grab the band with both hands and hold it at approximately chest high and close to your body.
2. There should be a little band resistance, but it should be easy to hold.
3. Engage your glutes and core. Don't overextend your back or overly tilt your hips.
4. Press the band directly out front in a straight line.
5. Extend your elbows fully as the band resistance increases.
6. The band will attempt to pull you toward it. Your spine will want to twist and your hips collapse. Don't let them.
7. Hold here for the duration of the set (20-40 seconds or as described in your training plan), trying to breath as you brace your core hard.
8. Reset and repeat on the other side.

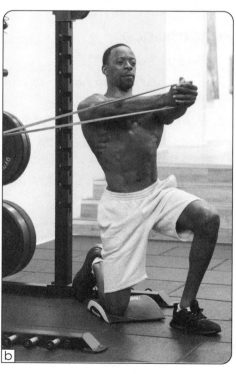

Tips for Success

- If you don't have access to much equipment, then the half-kneeling band isometric hold is a good training option that can be done almost anywhere.
- Progress to a heavier resistance band over time.

11
CABLE ANTICHOP

Level: Intermediate

Cable antichops develop stability from a half-kneeling position. As you chop the cable across your body, there's a demand for your core to stabilize your spine and hips under different conditions. Each position of the cable presents a unique challenge. At the same time you're resisting spinal rotation and lateral flexion, you're also working hard to keep your pelvis from tilting in multiple directions and your hips from shifting. Cable antichops can be performed at all levels and are a staple exercise for spinal health and core stability when performed correctly.

Setup

- Set a cable so it's near head height when you're standing. Attach a single D-handle or use a rope attachment.
- Position yourself approximately 10 inches (25 cm) away from the cable stack with the cable to one side.
- Get into a half-kneeling stance with your cable-side leg forward and opposite leg back.
- Bend both knees to 90-degree angles, and keep your torso upright.

Performance

1. Grab the cable.
2. Keep your core engaged, and maintain a stable half-kneeling position throughout.
3. Without twisting or hiking a hip to one side, chop the cable down toward the side of your back leg.
4. Keep the cable close to your body and bend your elbows as you swipe down across your torso.
5. When the cable has reached the bottom position in front of your thigh, reverse the movement, allowing the cable to return to the start position overhead.
6. Do not allow your torso or hips to change position.
7. Exhale as you press the cable down in front.
8. Inhale as you return the cable to its starting point.

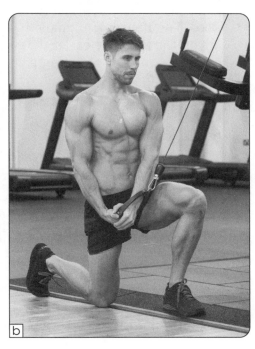

Tips for Success

- Cable antichops can be done in many positions—for example, standing, staggered, or a half-squat stance.
- A half-kneeling setup is a good starting point for learning how to resist lumbar extension and an anteriorly tilted pelvis. This is sometimes referred to as a scissored posture (ribs up, pelvis down).

12
SUSPENSION FALLOUT

Level: Advanced

Suspension fallouts are an advanced core exercise. They demand high levels of core engagement to resist spinal extension and an anterior tilt of your pelvis when in the bottom fallout position. Some people show impressive mastery of this exercise by reaching fully out in front while standing on their toes, almost looking like Superman at the finish. For most people, a good starting point is resisting the fall forward from your knees. The instability of the suspension trainer adds to the difficulty of this long-lever body position.

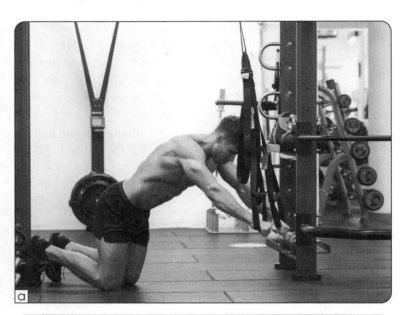

Setup

- Adjust the handles of your suspension trainer so they are 6 to 10 inches (15-25 cm) off the floor. The higher the handles are off the floor, the easier the exercise, so vary the height according to your level.

- Begin on all fours in front of the suspension trainer with your hands gripping the handles.

- The straps should be vertical as you hold them. Again, this can vary according to your level and the feel of the exercise.

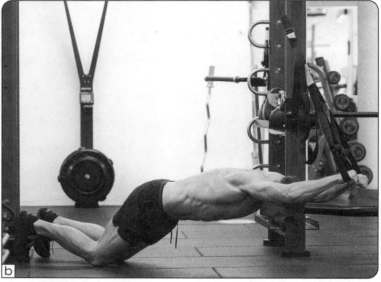

Performance

1. Brace your core and begin to drop your hips.

2. Push the straps of the suspension trainer in front of you, keeping your elbows straight as you do so.

3. Let your hips sink as far down and your arms to reach as far overhead as your core strength allows. If your back begins to cave or you feel pain, then you've gone too far.

4. Return to the start position using your core strength and a straight-arm pull-down.

5. Keep your head down and in a neutral position.

6. Maintain tension on the suspension trainer throughout; don't let it go slack at any point.

7. Breathe out on the lowering phase, and breathe in as you rise to the top.

Tips for Success

- You can load suspension fallouts by using a weighted vest.
- For an even more advanced variation that requires full-body strength, do the entire movement on your toes rather than your knees.

13
BEAR SHOULDER TAP

Level: Intermediate

Bear shoulder taps require you to hold strict 90-degree angles in your ankles, knees, hips, and shoulders while resisting spinal and pelvic rotation and extension. This is a highly challenging core exercise that has many variations to make it even more taxing.

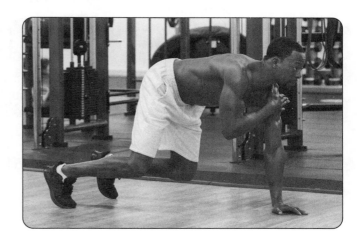

Setup

- Begin on the floor in a quadruped position (on all fours).
- Place your feet just wider than shoulder-width apart, similar to a typical squat stance.
- Place your hands shoulder-width apart and stacked under your shoulders.
- Keep your back and head neutral.

Performance

1. In a quadruped position, lift your knees just off the floor to resemble a squat that's been flipped horizontally.
2. Your knees should hover an inch or two (2.5-5 cm) off the floor, and your hands and toes are pressed firmly down.
3. With your back and neck neutral, engage your core at all times.
4. While maintaining a stable "bear" position, raise one hand off the floor, working hard to keep from dropping your hips or twisting your spine.
5. Tap your opposite shoulder, and then return your hand to the floor.
6. Repeat on the opposite side.
7. Your hips and spine should remain stable throughout.

Tips for Success

- Several core exercises can be performed in the bear position.
- In one variation, instead of tapping your opposite shoulder, use your lifted hand to transfer a stack of weight plates from one side to the other and then back again.
- Be creative in the use of your hands and feet in this position as long as you remember that the main goal is to maintain a stable pelvis and spine.

14
DEAD-STOP AB WHEEL ROLLOUT

Level: Advanced

Ab wheel rollouts are one of the most effective exercises for both core and abdominal training. Unique characteristics make them useful for performance, injury prevention, and aesthetic goals. How you perform the exercise can change the emphasis to each of these goals. As you lower, your core is working hard

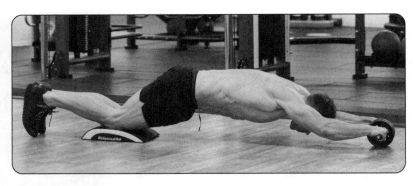

to resist spinal extension and an anterior tilt of your pelvis—the saggy back you often see in beginners to this exercise. As you reach the bottom, your core needs to work even harder to brake so you don't fall to the floor. This requires tremendous eccentric core strength. In a typical ab wheel rollout, you'd come back up immediately once you reach the bottom. But in the dead-stop ab wheel rollout, you add a static hold at the bottom. This requires isometric core strength and also makes it more difficult to come back up (because you can no longer use the muscles' elastic properties, and you need to overcome the inertia of the dead stop). The dead-stop ab wheel rollout develops both static and dynamic core strength using an antiextension movement pattern.

Setup

- You need an ab wheel and a foam pad or exercise mat for knee comfort; the pad or mat is optional.
- Position yourself on all fours, holding the ab wheel out in front.
- Keep your knees on the pad or mat throughout. They act as a pivot point.
- Pinch your glutes together and brace your core.

Performance

1. Push the ab roller forward, allowing your hips to drop with it.
2. Keep your back from overextending as you lower by engaging your core and glutes.
3. Reach the roller as far forward as you can with your arms fully overhead.
4. Pause in the deepest position for a two-second count.
5. Return to the top by pulling with your abdominals and driving your arms down.
6. As the roller reaches about level with your shoulders, you may flex your spine as if to perform a crunch, or you may keep it neutral.

Tips for Success

- The dead-stop ab wheel rollout can be performed with a flexed spine at the top or with a more neutral spine.
- Performing the exercise with a flexed spine increases the activation of your rectus abdominis, making it more of a six-pack exercise.
- Performing the exercise with a neutrally held spine promotes isometric strength and core stability.

15
BARBELL AB ROLLOUT

Level: Advanced

The barbell ab rollout, much like other roll-out variations, are one of the best exercises for working your core and developing six-pack abs. As you roll the barbell forward, your abdominals and core eccentrically resist lumbar extension and

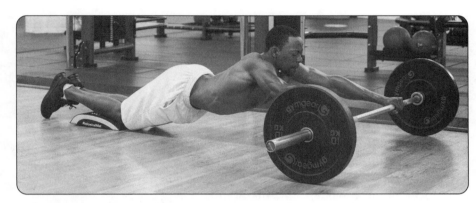

pelvic tilt. With a brief stop at the bottom, your core must engage hard before helping you return to the top. When you reach the top, your spine can remain neutral or you can accentuate spinal flexion to get a little more out of your abs.

Setup

- Place a few small round plates onto a barbell and use collars so they don't slide off.
- Use a foam pad or exercise mat for knee comfort (optional).
- Position yourself on all fours, holding the bar on the floor in front of your knees.
- Keep your knees on the pad or mat throughout; the knees act as a pivot point.
- Pinch your glutes together, and brace your core hard.

Performance

1. Push the barbell forward, allowing your hips to drop with it.
2. Engage your abs and glutes throughout in order to prevent an overly extended back.
3. Roll the barbell as far forward as you can. If you feel this in your lower back, then you've gone too far.
4. Depending on your range of motion and how wide the weight plates are, lower your nose as close to the floor as possible.
5. To come back up, pull your arms straight down toward your hips, dragging the barbell back toward you.
6. As the barbell reaches about level with your shoulders, you may either flex your spine into a crunchlike position at the top or keep your spine neutral.

Tips for Success

- The barbell ab rollout is an advanced exercise that many people try to progress by using more weight on the bar. While this works to some extent, it is not the most effective way to add progression.
- Instead, consider doing these while wearing a weighted vest.
- You may also attach a resistance band between the barbell and something sturdy in front of it. The band will pull you forward and load you more as you pull farther in.

16
SINGLE-ARM FRONT PLANK ON STABILITY BALL

Level: Hardcore

Performing a front plank on a stability ball creates an unstable environment. Put the basic front plank on a stability ball and take one arm off it, and you have a pretty hardcore exercise. Most of the instability from the ball directly affects the joints closest to it. So in this case, your shoulders receive a large effect, helping to recruit stabilizers around your shoulder girdle. This is on top of the instability added to the movement as a whole. This instability is further enhanced by lifting one arm off, which adds an antirotational component to the plank. You won't chisel your six-pack

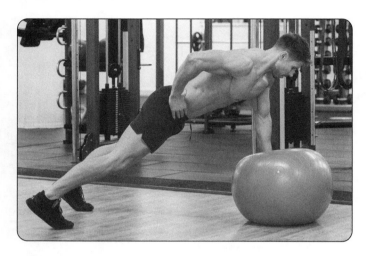

abs with this exercise, but you'll have a rock-solid midsection that'll be able to handle anything you throw at it.

Setup

- Use a small stability ball.
- Do not try this exercise until you first master foundational and intermediate plank variations.
- Position yourself in a basic front plank with both hands on the stability ball.

Performance

1. Engage your core and glutes throughout the exercise.
2. Maintaining spine and pelvic stability, carefully bring one hand slightly toward the center of the ball.
3. Lift the opposite hand, and either let it hover or move it back by your side.
4. Hold this position on one arm for the duration of the timed set, 10 to 30 seconds.
5. Do not let your hips drop or rotate.
6. As soon as you become too unstable, carefully dismount the stability ball.

Tips for Success

For more stability, push the stability ball against a wall. This will enable you to practice the position before the training wheels come off and the ball is able to roll in any direction.

17
MEDICINE BALL WALKOUT

Level: Advanced

Medicine ball walkouts are a novel way to train the antiextension core movement pattern. Using your hands to walk a medicine ball in front of you offers a unique demand to your shoulders, lats, core, and hips. These require very little equipment and are a good alternative to ab rollout variations.

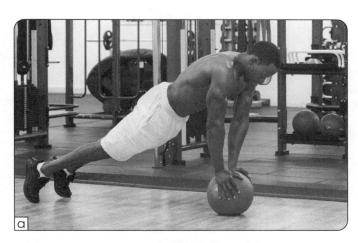

Setup

- Start in the basic front-plank position with both hands on a medicine ball.
- Place your feet shoulder-width apart.
- Align the hips, back, spine, and head.
- Engage the core and pinch the glutes together.

Performance

1. Initiate the movement by walking the medicine ball forward.
2. Keep your core and glutes engaged and your spine and head neutral.
3. Walk the ball forward as far as you can. If you begin to feel it in your lower back, then you've gone too far.

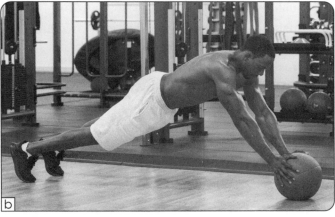

4. Walk the ball back to the start position under your shoulders.
5. One repetition consists of fully walking the ball out and back in.

Tips for Success

- For an intermediate option, perform medicine ball walkouts on your knees. Your hips should be fully extended.
- For a challenge, do these from a standing start.

18
STABILITY BALL ROLLOUT

Level: Foundational

Stability ball rollouts are a foundational exercise performed in much the same way as an ab wheel rollout. The difference, though, is that the larger size of the stability ball reduces range of motion and makes the roll forward easier for your core to control. These can be used as a regression of ab wheel rollouts, where you can build strength by increasing range of motion over time.

Setup

- You need a stability ball. The smaller the ball, the higher the difficulty.
- Use a foam pad or exercise mat for knee comfort (optional).
- Position yourself on all fours with your forearms on the stability ball in front.
- Squeeze your glutes and brace your core hard.

Performance

1. Push the stability ball forward, allowing your head to drop toward it and your hips to drop.
2. Push the ball as far forward as you can manage, ideally to where your hips are fully straightened and your arms are fully overhead.
3. Prevent your back from overextending by keeping your core and glutes engaged throughout.
4. Return to the top by using your abdominals, flexing your hips, and pulling your elbows in.
5. Exhale as you lower, and inhale as you return to the start position.

Tips for Success

- Stability rollouts can shift from a foundational exercise to a more advanced one in an instant.
- Perform stability ball rollouts on your toes instead of your knees for a real challenge. These somewhat resemble the slider body saw exercise.

19
HAMSTRING-ACTIVATED ROLLOUT

Level: Advanced

The hamstring-activated rollout relies on a phenomenon referred to as *reciprocal inhibition*. Quite simply, by activating your hamstrings you can "switch off" your hip flexors, thereby forcing your abdominals to work harder. You can encourage hamstring activation in various ways, but the easiest is by using a medicine ball behind your knees. The medicine ball is squeezed using your

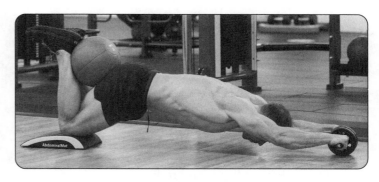

hamstrings, which inhibits your hip flexors. This exercise takes a big jump in difficulty, so be sure to master the dead-stop ab wheel rollout, barbell ab rollout, and stability ball rollout before attempting this exercise.

Setup

- You need an ab wheel, a foam pad or an exercise mat for knee comfort, and a medicine ball; the pad or mat is optional.
- Place the medicine ball behind your knees, squeezing it between your calves and hamstrings.
- Position yourself on all fours, holding the ab wheel out in front.
- Pinch your glutes together and brace your core hard.

Performance

1. Use your hamstrings to squeeze the medicine ball between your calves and hamstrings. If you can't do this, you may require a larger medicine ball.
2. Push the ab roller forward, allowing your hips to drop with it.
3. Reach as far forward with the roller as you can; your arms are fully extended overhead.
4. Engage your glutes and core throughout the exercise, and prevent your lower back from overextending. Squeezing the medicine ball makes this more difficult.
5. Return to the top by pulling with your abdominals and driving your arms straight down.
6. It's important to activate your hamstrings by squeezing the ball the entire time.
7. As the roller reaches about level with your shoulders, flex your spine as if to perform a crunch. Alternatively, you may keep your spine neutral throughout.

Tips for Success

- Hamstring-activated rollouts are an advanced exercise. To make them easier, revert to more basic rollouts.
- If you require even greater difficulty, then perform these wearing a weighted vest or adding isometric holds at the bottom of each rep.

20
STABILITY BALL KNEE TUCK TO ROLLOUT

Level: Advanced

Individually, stability ball knee tucks and stability ball rollouts are some of the best core exercises. This is based on the levels of muscle activation you can achieve with them. So combine them, and you have the ultimate dream team. The stability ball knee tuck to rollout isn't for beginners or if balance is a challenge. But if you have already mastered both knee tucks and rollouts as individual exercises, then take your core training to the next level with this advanced antiextension exercise.

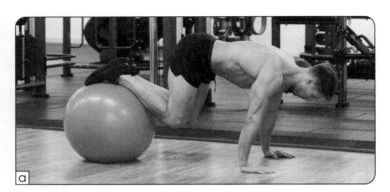

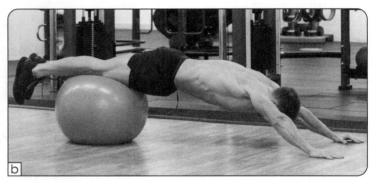

Setup

- Place your hands on the floor and both feet on a stability ball.
- Roll the stability ball so that your shins rest on it. Adjust this depending on how high or low on your shins feels best.
- Engage your core throughout and keep your spine neutral or with very slight flexion.

Performance

1. This is a two-part exercise starting with the knee-tuck portion.
2. Pull your knees in toward your chest, allowing the ball to roll along your shins in a straight line.
3. Bring your knees up to a point just beyond level with the crease of your hips. This will cause a slight tucking of your pelvis.
4. Return the ball back to the start, ensuring your back or hips do not drop.
5. Once you are back to the start position, push your hands into the floor so you continue to roll the ball up your shins. At this point, the stability ball should be close to your knees and your arms overhead. This is the rollout portion.
6. Pull back to the start position so that your shoulders are over your wrists and the stability ball is at rest under your lower shins.
7. This is one complete repetition.

Tips for Success

You can also do the knee tuck to rollout using a suspension trainer or even core sliders. These can make it more difficult to resist extension, but they are easier from a stability standpoint.

21
SLIDER BODY SAW

Level: Advanced

The slider body saw is an advanced exercise used to train the antiextension pattern. Body saws work more than just the front of your abs and core. They are one of the best exercises to chisel your obliques, too. Slider body saws offer an advanced exercise to work your entire core to the max.

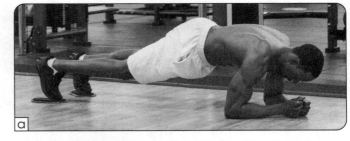

Setup

- Begin in a basic front plank with your feet on core sliders.
- Place your elbows on a mat or foam pad for comfort (optional).
- Brace your core (imagine 360 degrees of air around your spine, and contract your abdominals), and pinch your glutes together to stabilize your spine and pelvis.

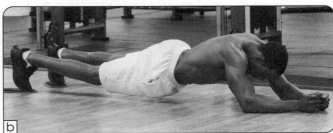

Performance

1. Begin by using your elbows and forearms to push your head away from your fists.
2. Your entire body should travel backward as one strong unit, made possible with the core sliders gliding along the floor.
3. Slide back as far as you're capable of, ensuring your core is engaged and spine and hips are stable.
4. Use your elbows and forearms to pull back to the start position, which resembles a basic front plank.

Tips for Success

Slider body saws are easier said than done. However, if you have a core made of steel and want to progress these, wearing a weighted vest is the best way.

22
SLIDER PUSH-UP REACH

Level: Advanced

Push-ups can be seen as moving planks. They require core strength and stability, which allows an efficient push away from the floor. The slider push-up reach incorporates an anti-rotational component to the moving plank, while working out your chest, shoulders, and arms at the same time. This is made possible by reaching the arm forward as you lower into the push-up. If you're ready for an advanced push-up variation, then these offer a highly efficient way to hit your core and upper body at the same time.

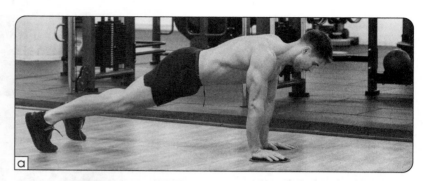

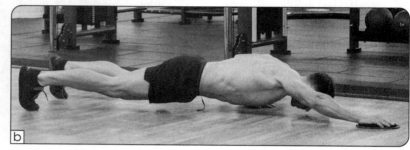

Setup

- Begin in a push-up position with one hand placed firmly on a core slider.
- Keep your core and glutes engaged and spine and pelvis stable throughout.

Performance

1. Lower into a full push-up while pushing the slider along the floor so that one arm is reaching overhead.
2. Attempt to achieve full range of motion by touching your nose to the floor.
3. Resist the urge to rotate your pelvis.
4. Return to the top of the push-up by pressing through the bent arm and sliding the other hand back to the start under your shoulder.
5. Perform all of your repetitions on one side before repeating on the other.

Tips for Success

- Slider push-ups can be performed with two core sliders and alternating arms.
- You may also challenge your rotational stability by reaching out toward the side instead of overhead.

23
PUSH-UP WITH LOAD OVER HIPS

Level: Intermediate

Push-ups are a time-efficient way to work on your plank position while also getting in a great upper-body workout. While there are many ways to increase the difficulty of push-ups for your upper body, there aren't many ways to increase the intensity (load) to work your core harder. Push-ups are antiextension exercises that engage your core in order to resist spinal extension and an anterior tilt of your pelvis. Placing a load over your hips is one way to make push-ups work your core harder.

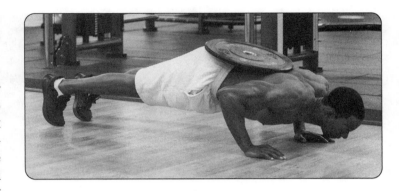

Setup

- You need a weight plate or other form of load to place over your hips.
- Begin in a standard push-up position.
- Place the load over your hips, or ask a partner to do it.
- The load should be centered at about the level of your sacrum (just above your tailbone).
- Engage your glutes and core to prevent the load from pulling you into lumbar extension and anteriorly tilting the pelvis.

Performance

1. Lower into the full push-up position, maintaining alignment between your head, shoulders, spine, and hips.
2. Engage your core throughout because the load challenges it even more.
3. Full range of motion is achieved when your nose touches the floor.
4. "Push the floor away" to return to the top of the push-up. Do not overly round your shoulders.
5. Inhale as you lower, and exhale as you push the floor away.
6. When the set is finished, remove the weight or ask a partner to do it for you.

Tips for Success

- If you see any push-up variation as a moving plank, you'll never do a bad push-up again.
- If you have access to them, try chains over your hips. The swinging effect adds instability. It's also a comfortable way to add resistance.

24
ECCENTRIC ONE-ARM PUSH-UP

Level: Advanced

One-arm push-ups require tremendous upper-body strength when done correctly. Sure, they're a great party trick, but for them to do you some good, you also need to hold a strict form and level hips. The eccentric one-arm push-up is easier to perform than a strict one-arm push-up, but it offers the same benefits to your core strength. Use eccentric one-arm push-ups to build upper body strength and an unbreakable core!

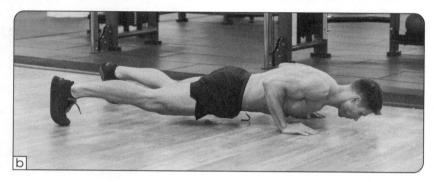

Setup

- Begin in a basic push-up position but with your feet a little wider to start off.
- Take one hand off the floor and allow it to hover, ready to catch you as you lower.
- Keep your core and glutes engaged, and resist the rotation in your hips.

Performance

1. Using just one arm, lower yourself in a controlled manner. If you have sufficient upper-body strength, you should be able to lower to within a few inches of the floor.
2. Take three or four seconds to fully lower.
3. Maintain a strong core and stable spine and hips.
4. When you reach the lowest point that your strength allows, place the free hand on the floor under your shoulder.
5. Press back to the top of the push-up using both hands. This will be significantly easier.
6. Perform all of your repetitions on one side before switching to the other.

Tips for Success

- Eccentric one-arm push-ups place a significant eccentric load through your upper body, making these an effective bodybuilding exercise for your chest, shoulders, and triceps, as well as benefitting your overall core strength.
- To make these a little easier, do them with your hands on a box or bench. The higher the box or bench, the easier these will be.
- Work down to being able to do them on the floor with a full range of motion over time.

25
ONE-ARM CABLE ANTIPRESS

Level: Intermediate

Your ability to press and punch with one arm often isn't limited by the strength of your upper body. Instead it is very much reliant on your antirotational core strength. In a standing position, force is mostly generated from your hips and travels through your core in a whipping motion. On the other hand, limiting the whip from your lower body requires tremendous core stability to hold a static pelvis and spine. This static position is the base from which you press. The one-arm cable antipress is a highly functional exercise that builds core strength and athleticism.

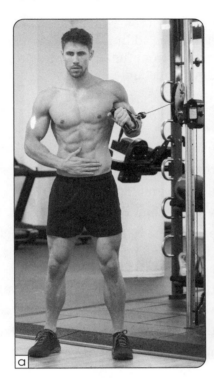 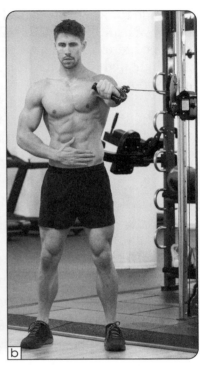

Setup

- Place a D-handle on a cable, and set it at about shoulder height.
- Grab the cable so that it is aligned outside of your elbow.
- Face your torso directly away from the stack and to one side.
- Slightly soften your knees, and keep your torso upright.
- Place your nonworking arm on your hip.
- Brace your core and "spread the floor" with your feet to engage your glutes.

Performance

1. Maintaining trunk stability, press the cable directly in front with one arm.
2. As you press, your spine and hips will want to rotate. Resist and don't allow movement to take place apart from that of the pressing arm.
3. Press the cable out fully until your elbow is extended. Exhale as you do so.
4. Return the cable to its starting point toward your shoulder. Inhale as you do.
5. Perform all repetitions on one side before switching to the other side.

Tips for Success

- The one-arm cable antipress doesn't have to be a press in a horizontal direction.
- Depending on your emphasis, you can set the cable a little lower and press at an incline angle, or set the cable higher and press downward a little more.
- You can use staggered, kneeling, and half-kneeling stances, too. To emphasize the core, resist spine and pelvic movement while pressing from these positions.

26
RENEGADE ROW

Level: Intermediate

Renegade rows combine a push-up with a row while holding a basic front plank. They build antiextension and antirotational strength while adding fun and variety to your training. They are a highly efficient exercise, but to get the most from them for your core, you need to keep the reps honest. Start light and focus on controlling spine and pelvic motion before increasing the weight for more upper-body and back focus.

Setup

- Place two dumbbells on the floor. Hex-shaped dumbbells work best.
- Position yourself in a basic front plank, and grip the dumbbells under your shoulders.
- Align your head, shoulders, spine, and hips.
- Begin with a stance slightly wider than shoulder width.
- Engage your core and glutes to resist rotation in each dumbbell row.

Performance

1. Maintaining stability throughout, row one dumbbell in toward your chest.
2. Do not allow your hips to twist. If they do, widen your stance or use a lighter weight.
3. Return the dumbbell straight to the floor, and then immediately repeat on the other side.
4. Exhale as you pull the dumbbell in toward your chest.
5. Inhale as you return the dumbbell to the floor.

Tips for Success

There are many ways to perform renegade rows. For example, try incorporating push-ups, squats, or deadlifts in to them if you need to maximize time efficiency and for a full-body workout.

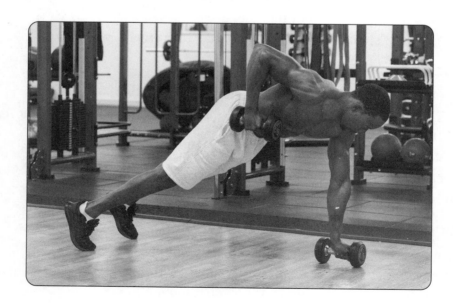

27
PLANK CABLE ROW

Level: Intermediate

The plank cable row combines a pulling action (think pull-downs and pull-ups, but horizontally) with a basic front plank. This combination exercise requires you to hold your spine and pelvis stable while forces try to twist and extend your spine. This is a good choice for maximizing training efficiency and saving time.

Setup

- Set a cable attached to a D-handle to a low position.
- Get into a basic front plank position in front of the cable. Your head should point toward the cable. Make sure you have enough space to row using a full range of motion.
- Keep your head, shoulders, spine, and hips aligned throughout, and don't allow your hips to rotate.
- Start with a wide stance with your feet, narrowing it as you progress.
- Grab the D-handle.

Performance

1. Maintaining a stable front-plank position, row the cable in toward your shoulder. Pull your thumb to your arm pit.
2. As you row, resist spine and pelvic movement.
3. Reverse the row to the start position while maintaining trunk stability.

Tips for Success

The plank cable row can also be done using a resistance band as part of a minimal-equipment workout.

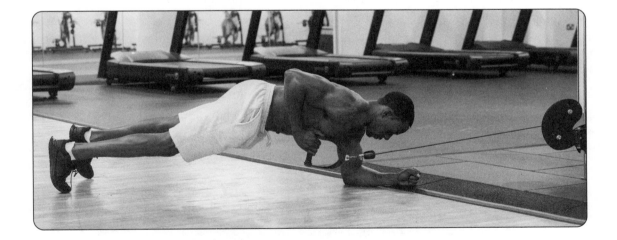

28
PLANK KETTLEBELL PRESS

Level: Advanced

The plank kettlebell press is an advanced core exercise that combines a plank with a kettlebell press (similar to a shoulder press, but horizontal). The position of the kettlebell makes the press harder, even when a light weight is used. It also requires sufficient shoulder mobility. Use the plank kettlebell press to develop bulletproof core and shoulders.

Setup

- Get into a basic front-plank position.
- Align your head, shoulders, spine, and hips.
- Grip a very light kettlebell in one hand as if to press overhead.
- Engage your core and glutes.

Performance

1. Firmly grip the kettlebell and ensure it is resting comfortably against your forearm.
2. Maintaining the basic front-plank position, press the kettlebell forward until your arm is fully extended.
3. Resist rotation of your hips and don't overextend your spine.
4. Bring the kettlebell immediately back in toward your shoulder.
5. Perform the repetitions on one side before switching to the other.

Tips for Success

- The plank kettlebell press also doubles as a shoulder strengthener and stabilizer.
- For an unstable challenge, hold your opposite foot off the floor—for example, press with your right arm while your left leg is off the floor.
- For an easier alternative that still challenges your core, perform the movement with your knees on the floor.

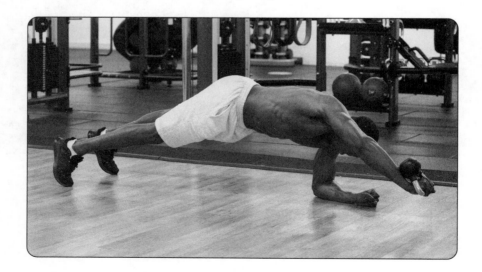

29
PLANK WHILE STACKING PLATES

Level: Intermediate

Setup
- Begin with three small weight plates stacked on top of each other on the floor.
- Position yourself in a basic-front plank with the stacked plates just outside one of your planted elbows.

Performance
1. With the hand next to the stacked plates, pick up one plate.
2. Lift the plate over your back, and place it in the groove of your lower back.
3. Your spine should be neutral and your head, shoulders, spine, and hips aligned throughout the movement.
4. Repeat the process until all of the plates are stacked on your back or they fall off, failing the challenge.
5. Remove the plates one at a time with the other hand, stacking them on the opposite side.

Tips for Success
- To make this exercise easier, use plastic cones.
- If you have limited equipment or you are at home, stacking books on your back is a fun challenge.
- To increase difficulty, stack heavier weight plates.

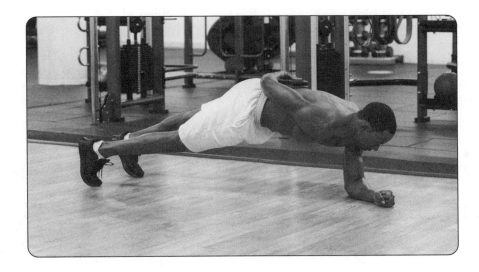

30
BASIC DEAD BUG

Level: Foundational

The basic dead bug is a staple exercise to improve foundational core strength. Lying on your back on the floor with feet lifted off the floor, your spine is kept stable while your arms and legs move contralaterally. Lifting and lowering your arms and legs in opposition increases the demand for your core to resist spinal and pelvic rotation. Spinal extension is also being challenged. The coordination and strength developed through this exercise are highly applicable to human locomotion, walking, and sprinting. For this reason, it's often used in rehabilitation settings as well as the programs of elite athletes to build functional core strength.

Setup

- Lie on your back on the floor with arms extended and pointing to the sky.
- Bend your hips and knees to 90-degree angles.
- Brace your core and imagine pressing your lower back into the floor. A small towel between your lower back and the floor can sometimes help by adding comfort and improving spinal awareness.

Performance

1. Start by taking a deep breath in.
2. Exhale and slowly extend one leg toward the floor, making the leg as long as you can.
3. At the same time, bring your opposite arm fully overhead.
4. Fully brace your core and resist spinal or pelvic motion.
5. Slowly return the arm and leg to the starting position.
6. Repeat with the opposite arm and leg for the desired number of repetitions.

Tips for Success

The best way to load the basic dead bug is to attach small weights to the ankles and wrists. Alternatively, you may attach weights to your ankles and hold very small dumbbells in your hands. Even the lightest weights can feel like a big difference.

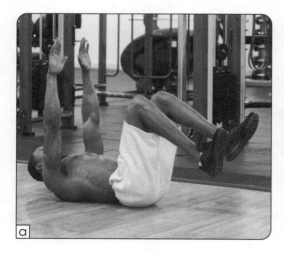
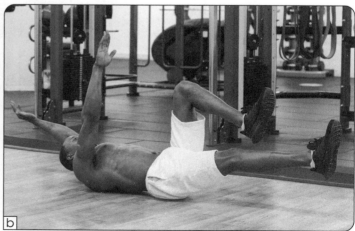

31
DEAD BUG CRUSHING MEDICINE BALL

Level: Intermediate

Increase the demands on your core during a basic dead bug by adding a medicine ball. In this exercise, you "crush" the medicine ball between your elbow and the opposite knee. This encourages spinal flexion and a hard contraction of your anterior core muscles. It's a good way to strengthen the contralateral shoulder-to-hip pattern that dead bugs target so effectively.

Setup

- You need a light medicine ball. A small stability ball also works as does a soccer ball or basketball if you have sufficient hip flexion mobility.
- Lie on your back on the floor with arms extended and pointing to the sky.
- Bend your hips and knees to 90-degree angles.
- Place the ball between your elbow and opposite knee. Squeeze it hard so it doesn't move and to increase activation of your abdominals.
- Brace your core and imagine pressing your lower back into the floor.

Performance

1. Start by taking a deep breath in.
2. Exhale and slowly extend your free leg toward the floor, making it as long as you can. The free leg is the one that isn't in contact with the ball.
3. At the same time, bring your free arm fully overhead.
4. The ball should remain crushed between the opposing elbow and knee.
5. Slowly return the arm and leg to the starting point.
6. Repeat on the same side for the desired number of repetitions.
7. Place the ball between the other arm and leg and repeat.

Tips for Success

For an even more advanced variation, perform these on a flat bench. This will increase instability, making it more difficult to keep the ball in place.

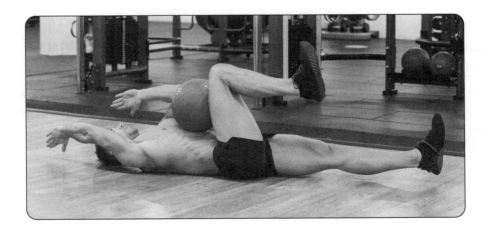

32
BASIC CABLE PALLOF PRESS

Level: Intermediate

Basic cable Pallof presses are a go-to exercise for developing antirotational core strength and stability. They are easily scalable and have many beginner and advanced variations. They have great application to injury rehabilitation, training for strength and power athletes, and functional fitness. As a bonus, Pallof presses put you in a perfect position to incorporate breathing drills, too. Try this basic variation before attempting slightly more advanced versions, such as the Dead Bug Pallof Press for example.

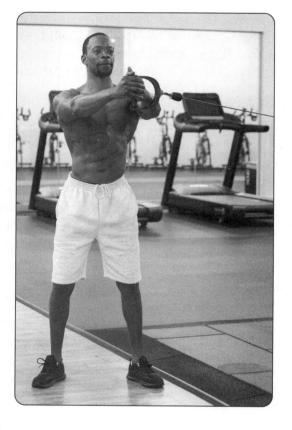

Setup

- The basic cable Pallof press begins from a standing position.
- Attach a D-handle to a cable set to about chest height.
- Stand with one side toward the cable in a soft stance, feet about shoulder-width apart, and the cable in both hands held to the center of your chest.

Performance

1. Brace your core, and imagine spreading the floor with your feet to activate your glutes.
2. Keep your shoulders back and head facing forward.
3. Press the cable away from your chest and keep it central. As you push it farther away from your body, the resistance coming from one side will make it harder to resist twisting.
4. Press out as far as possible.
5. Maintain whole-body tension and hold for 10 seconds to complete one repetition.
6. Release the resistance by bringing the cable in and taking a breath.
7. Repeat for the desired number of 10-second intervals.

Tips for Success

- Pallof presses can be performed for a continuous period of time (for example, 30 seconds). However, this is difficult, it makes it hard to breathe, and technique deteriorates.
- Instead, splitting the holds into 10-second intervals allows the quality to remain high throughout. For example, if your goal is to hold for 30 seconds, then do three 10-second reps for a higher-quality set.
- Several ways to perform Pallof presses include standing stance, half-kneeling stance, staggered stance, athletic stance, tall-kneeling stance, seated, vertical, and drawing letters and numbers with the cable while holding it. See table 10.1 for additional variations.

Table 10.1 Pallof Press Variations

	Basic cable	Basic band	Cable overhead	Band overhead	Cable overhead from behind	Band overhead from behind
Tall standing	✓	✓				
Athletic stance	✓	✓	✓	✓	✓	✓
Sumo stance	✓	✓	✓	✓	✓	✓
Squat stance	✓	✓	✓	✓	✓	✓
Tall split stance	✓	✓	✓	✓	✓	✓
Low split stance	✓	✓	✓	✓	✓	✓
Tall kneeling	✓	✓	✓	✓		
Half kneeling	✓	✓	✓	✓	✓	✓
Narrow half kneeling	✓	✓			✓	✓

Although it is possible to perform a variation using equipment that is not checked, those variations aren't as effective as the ones that are checked.

33
DEAD BUG PALLOF PRESS

Level: Intermediate

Individually, the basic dead bug and the Pallof press variations are highly effective core exercises. While dead bugs are primarily antiextension and antirotational core exercises, Pallof presses put you in an ideal position to train the antirotation pattern even more. Combine the basic dead bug with a Pallof press, and you have a powerful core combination.

Setup

- Place a D-handle on a cable and set it to a height approximately an arm's length from the floor. Adjust the height depending on what feels best to you.
- Lie on your back on the floor with one side toward the cable.
- Grab the cable and hold it to your chest. The cable and your torso should form an approximately 90-degree angle.
- Bend your hips and knees to 90-degree angles.
- Brace your core and imagine pressing your lower back into the floor.
- Do not let the cable pull you toward it. For that reason, start light and build from there.

Performance

1. Take a deep breath, brace your core, and press the cable directly toward the sky and away from your chest.
2. Keep the cable down the midline of your body with arms fully extended.

3. Exhale and slowly extend one leg toward the floor, making it as long as you can.

4. Resist all movement except that of your moving leg.

5. Slowly return the leg to the starting position and repeat on the other side.

6. Alternate sides while holding the Pallof press position with the cable.

Tips for Success

If the gym is busy or you're working out at home, perform this exercise using a resistance band.

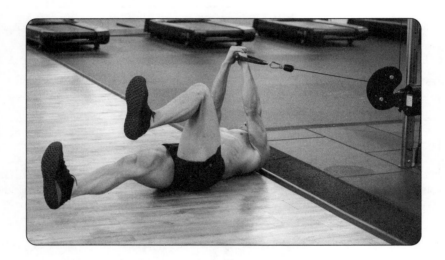

34
BANDED LEG LOWER

Level: Intermediate

Imagine you are lying on your back on the floor with both feet in the air and legs straight. Now lock one leg in place with a resistance band or something similar and lower the opposite leg. This one-leg-locked and other-leg-lowering action is a useful exercise for developing antirotational core strength. At the same time, it opens your hips, wakes up your core, and loosens your stiff hamstrings.

Setup

- Attach a band to a sturdy support approximately an arm's length from the floor.
- Lie on your back on the floor, gripping the band in both hands, and your arms extended toward the sky.
- Make sure you're far enough away to create tension in the band.
- Bend your hips to a 90-degree angle or as far as your flexibility allows with your knees fully straight.
- Dorsiflex your ankles (pull toes toward shins) and face the soles of your shoes toward the ceiling.
- Take a deep breath in and brace your core.

Performance

1. Pull the band down slightly with straight arms to engage your lats.

2. Press your lower back into the floor and keep your ribs down.

3. Exhale and slowly lower one leg toward the floor making the leg as long as you can.

4. Maintain band and lat tension, and keep the opposite leg lifted.

5. Fully brace your core, and resist spinal or pelvic motion.

6. Slowly return the leg to the starting point.

7. One leg remains locked at the top at all times while the other lowers and lifts, alternating on each side.

Tips for Success

- Banded leg lowers are a useful exercise to include in your core warm-up to get everything fired up and ready for action.
- As a warm-up exercise, go a little lighter and focus on awareness of your core and breathing.
- As a main exercise for maximal core engagement, go as heavy as you can handle.
- You can also do this exercise holding a cable with a rope attachment instead of a band.

35
BASIC BIRD DOG

Level: Foundational

The basic bird dog might sound like a made-up name, but it's a popular exercise among trainers and coaches for good reason. The basic bird dog puts you in a quadruped position (all fours) to strengthen your core, hips, back, and shoulders. There's more than meets the eye to this exercise because in addition to the antirotational core component, other areas are worked at the same time. By strengthening your glutes and hip abductors, improving your balance, and increasing your shoulder mobility, your entire body gets a great workout.

Setup

- Kneel on the floor on all fours with your knees directly under your hips and hands stacked directly under your shoulders.
- Your spine should be neutral and eyes looking to the floor.
- Brace your core; imagine 360 degrees of air around your spine while keeping your abdominals engaged.

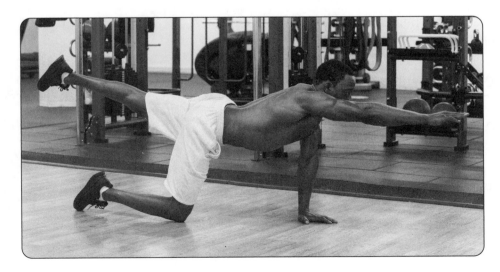

Performance

1. Begin by raising an arm and opposite leg at the same time.
2. Extend your clenched fist as far from your opposite foot as possible.
3. Engage your glutes to extend your hip and increase stability.
4. Do not overextend your lower back.
5. Resist rotation as your opposite arm and leg extend.
6. Bring your arm and leg back, and then repeat on the other side.

Tips for Success

For an advanced challenge, why not try the bird dog row? Simply perform the basic bird dog as described, but on a flat bench. Instead of your arm reaching forward, perform a row with a kettlebell or dumbbell in that hand. Keep the extended leg locked in its extended position while you row. Adding weight to this exercise requires tremendous core strength and stability.

36
LANDMINE RAINBOW

Level: Intermediate

Landmine training is all the rage and for good reason. The landmine, sometimes referred to as an angled barbell, offers another dimension to your full-body workouts. It has the ability to load certain movements in directions not offered with free weights or even cables. The landmine rainbow is one use for the landmine, and it trains the ability to resist rotation and lateral flexion.

Setup

- Place an empty barbell in a purpose-built landmine unit.
- Start without weight on the landmine as you practice the technique.
- Stand facing the landmine unit with the barbell in your hands and held to your chest.
- Soften your knees, and push your hips slightly back.

Performance

1. Press the barbell away from your chest, but keep your elbows slightly bent.

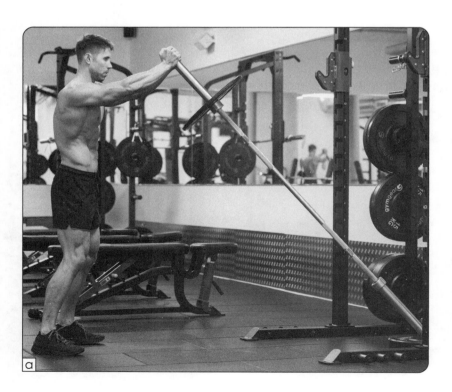

2. Brace your core and "spread the floor" with your stance to increase glute engagement.

3. Swipe the barbell from side to side across your body.

4. Move the bar from left to right using your arms while keeping the rest of your body static. The distance the bar is able to travel depends on your strength and body structure.

5. Resist hip and spinal movement throughout.

6. Once the set is over, the bar will return to the middle, to your chest, and then back to the floor.

7. Use a breathing pattern that feels comfortable; just breathing at all poses a challenge to many people.

Tips for Success

If you don't have a landmine unit, there are a few ways to set one up safely in any commercial gym. Here's one option (see photo). The bar rests in the hole of a plate. If you have one, you can also place a hexagonal dumbbell on top for additional safety.

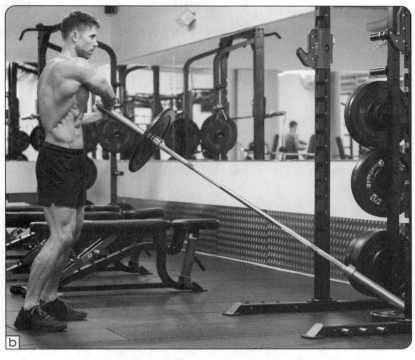

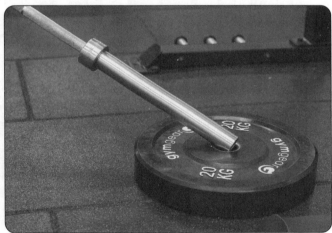

A makeshift landmine unit.

37
LANDMINE SQUAT RAINBOW

Level: Hardcore

The landmine squat rainbow is an extremely advanced exercise when done right. A left-to-right swipe of the landmine trains core stability in an antirotation and anti-lateral-flexion capacity. This is combined with the extra challenge of holding a squat position. This requires tremendous core and hip stability and lower-body isometric strength.

Setup

- Place an empty barbell in a purpose-built or makeshift landmine unit.
- Start without weight on the bar as you practice the technique.
- Stand facing the landmine unit with the barbell in your hands and held to your chest.
- Put some weight on your heels and sit into a squat with a 90-degree knee bend.

Performance

1. Press the barbell away from your chest, but keep your elbows slightly bent.

2. Hold the 90-degree squat position while starting to swipe the barbell from side to side across your body.

3. Resist hip or spinal movement throughout, and do not come out of the squat.

4. Once the set is over, the bar will return to the middle before you can stand up and out of the squat.

5. Use a breathing pattern that feels comfortable. This is a highly challenging exercise, and many people find breathing difficult.

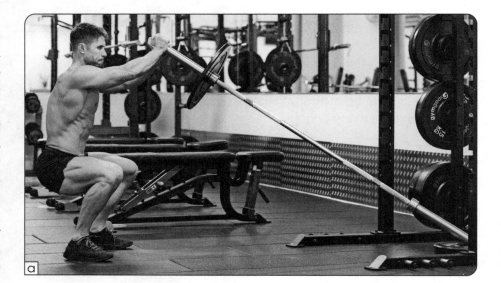

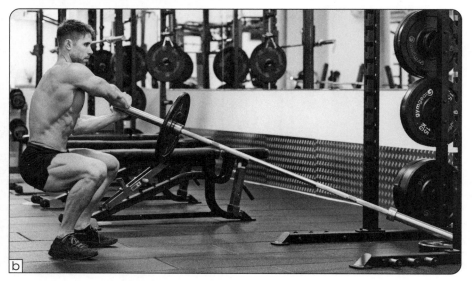

Tips for Success

The difficulty and challenge rating of this exercise are high. You might want to start with a half-squat before gradually lowering farther over time.

38

SUSPENSION PALLOF PRESS

Level: Intermediate

Pallof press variations are typically performed using cables, but you can use your own body weight to load them, too. Although in a Pallof press it's usually the cable stack that moves, during a suspension Pallof press, it's your own body that moves away from the suspension trainer. Holding a suspension trainer in front of you in the same way you would during a Pallof press requires a strong core to keep your body line from distorting. Resisting the temptation to drop your hips and twist your spine will allow you to build a solid core using just your own body weight.

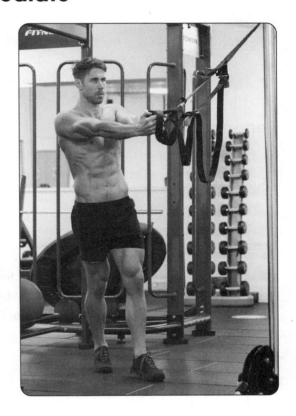

Setup

- In a split-stance position, face about 90-degrees away from the suspension trainer anchor. Your front leg should be on the same side as the anchor.
- Hold the suspension trainer level with your chest with extended arms.
- The suspension trainer should line up with the anchor point and your extended arm to form a 90-degree angle.

Performance

1. Holding the suspension trainer handles, begin to lean sideways and away from the anchor point.
2. Keep your arms extended and at chest level.
3. Your core should be maximally engaged at all times.
4. Maintaining this position, begin to pull the suspension trainer handle in toward your chest before pressing it out again.
5. Hold the pressed-out position for a few seconds each time.
6. Do not move any body part except your arms. Maintain whole-body stability throughout.

Tips for Success

- To increase difficulty, walk yourself farther in toward the anchor point of the suspension trainer.
- To make the suspension Pallof press easier, walk farther away from the anchor point. This means pressing the suspension trainer away from your chest while holding your torso at a more upright angle.

39
SUSPENSION OVERHEAD PALLOF PRESS

Level: Intermediate

The suspension overhead Pallof press uses your own body weight to train the anti-lateral-flexion movement pattern. This is made possible by holding your arms in an overhead position rather than straight out in front. The angle of your body can easily be manipulated to either increase or decrease the demand on your core to resist lateral flexion.

Setup

- From a split-stance position, face about 90 degrees away from the suspension trainer anchor. Your front leg should be on the same side as the anchor.
- Hold the suspension trainer on your chest with both hands with your knuckles facing upward and ready to press overhead.

Performance

1. Holding the suspension trainer handles, begin to lean sideways and away from the anchor point.
2. The suspension trainer should be close to your chest at this point.
3. Keep your core maximally engaged at all times.
4. Begin to press the suspension trainer handle directly overhead to form a straight line with your torso.
5. Take your arms fully overhead before holding here for a few seconds.
6. If the overhead position is too difficult to hold, then walk a little farther away from the suspension trainer anchor point to make it easier.
7. Resist dropping your hip and bending your spine laterally.
8. Bring the suspension trainer back in toward your chest, take a breath, and then go again.

Tips for Success

- Overhead Pallof presses also work well from a half-kneeling position with your back knee on the floor.
- Overhead Pallof presses may also be done using a cable.

Exercises to Complement Your Six-Pack Workout

Previous chapters have outlined exercises that work all functions of your abdominals and core. This information will allow you to blend the best exercises to not only build a six-pack that looks good but also performs well at the same time. While abdominal strength training and core strength training contribute to both form and function, in order to get the most from these exercises, you also need to ensure they are part of a bigger training picture—a picture that ensures your whole body is evenly balanced. This is what's referred to as being structurally balanced, and it is important if you want to build whole-body resistance to injury and to promote spinal health.

Your abs and anterior core muscles might look great after exploring all of the exercises in chapters 7 through 10, but you also need to think about muscles such as your glutes, spinal erectors, and adductors. The spinal erectors are essentially the muscles that keep your spine lined up. They are predominantly made up of slow twitch muscle fibers and can be thought of as more endurance-based. Although these muscles are often neglected, they are the ones that help further stabilize your lumbar, hip, and pelvic region.

Remember, staying injury free and healthy is important for aesthetics, too. If you're injured, then you miss training sessions. If you experience pain doing certain exercises, then you might have to avoid those exercises and won't receive their benefits. And let's not forget that if your body feels weak overall, and maybe a few areas aren't as strong as they once were, your overall activity levels will decline. When you burn less energy, you won't be able to do the work necessary to uncover your six-pack. You might not be concerned with injury prevention or maintaining whole-body structural balance right now, but you will be when they start to affect what you see in the mirror.

You don't need to spend much time on these exercises, but here are the top six you should include in your overall training plan to ensure structural balance. Variations of each exercise are offered, so you will have plenty of options to use throughout the year. With all of these exercises try to focus on getting a full-braced position with your core; imagining 360 degrees of air around your spine with your abdominals contracted. As far as breathing is concerned, do what feels best in order for this braced position to be achieved.

1
BARBELL HIP THRUST

Level: Intermediate

The barbell hip thrust is a popular exercise for developing and strengthening your glutes. Alongside glute bridge variations, these exercises are classified as bent-knee hip extension exercises. By bending your knees during hip extension, you reduce the amount of force that your hamstrings can produce, forcing your glutes to work as the primary hip extensors.

Because the bar is placed across your hips during hip thrusts and glute bridges, you will load the hip extension horizontally. This horizontal load vector has a great transfer to athletic movements. Load vector is when the direction in which you are producing force closely resembles such activities as sprinting and propelling yourself forward. This also loads your glutes efficiently in their fully shortened position. This leads to more tension and more muscle growth.

Unlike glute bridges, which take place on the floor, hip thrusts are performed with your back positioned on a step or bench. This allows your shins to remain vertical for a larger portion of the movement and for an increased range of motion. Because of the increased range of motion, you might find barbell glute bridging on the floor a better option if you struggle with hip-hinging mechanics. However, if you want to target and strengthen your glutes effectively, include hip thrusts in your training plan.

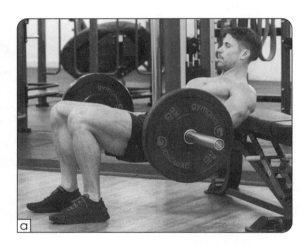

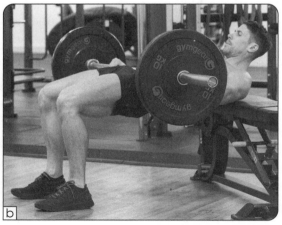

Setup

- Adjust the height of the bench or step according to what feels best.
- Position yourself so your shoulder blades are resting on the bench.
- Place your feet approximately hip-width apart and press your heels firmly into the floor.
- Roll a padded barbell across your hips. You can also use a foam pad for comfort.

Performance

1. Bend your knees to 90 degrees.
2. Tuck your chin.
3. Take a deep breath in and contract your abdominals and glutes before you initiate movement.
4. Push through your heels and extend your hips toward the ceiling.
5. Focus on a full contraction of your glutes at the top, and do not overextend your lower back.
6. Your shins should be vertical (perpendicular to the floor) when you reach the top.
7. Lower under control to just beyond the point that your shins are no longer vertical. There is nothing wrong with lowering farther; however, this shifts the emphasis to your hamstrings.
8. Exhale as you thrust upward, and inhale as you lower.

Variations

- Single-leg hip thrust
- Staggered-stance hip thrust
- Two-one method hip thrust (rise with both legs, and lower with one)
- Different loading options, including a dumbbell, sandbag, machine, resistance band, or chains across your hips

2
STABILITY BALL HAMSTRING CURL

Level: Intermediate

Stability ball hamstring curls are a good choice for strengthening your hamstrings and improving the health of your knees. When training your abdominals, it's common to also be strengthening your hip flexors a little at the same time—even if you might be trying to avoid this.

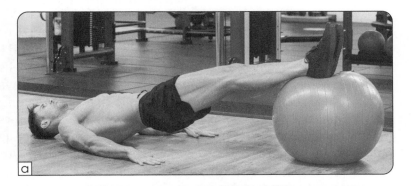

To maintain structural balance around the hips, consider the muscles around the backside, too. Strengthening your glutes and hamstrings alongside your core and abdominals creates a stronger and healthier spine.

Well-conditioned hamstrings help prevent hamstring injuries, too. If you have performance goals in mind, then stability ball hamstring curls will keep you healthy and on track. Using a stability ball is a versatile way to do hamstring curls, and the instability offers additional benefits.

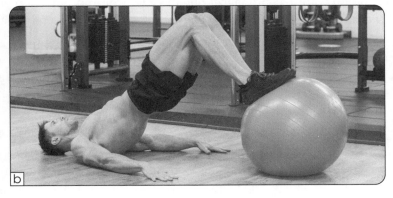

Setup

- Choose the right ball size based on your height and manufacturer instructions.
- Lie on your back on the floor or a mat (optional) with your heels on the ball.
- Place your hands on the floor by your side.

Performance

1. Push your hips up and squeeze your glutes to keep them extended.
2. Use your hamstrings to drag your heels toward your butt.
3. Stop the curl right before you lose tension in the hamstrings. Curling too far decreases the tension.
4. Slowly and under control, lower to the start position.
5. Keep your hips off the floor throughout.
6. Exhale as you curl in; inhale as you curl out.

Variations

- Stability ball single-leg hamstring curls
- Hamstring curl with core sliders
- Hamstring curl with a suspension trainer if you require more stability

---

3

45-DEGREE BACK EXTENSION

Level: Foundational

Back extensions are one of the most underappreciated exercises for strengthening your entire posterior chain, which includes your hamstrings, glutes, and lower back. Sometimes referred to as hyperextensions, they're often performed as their name implies using a technique that encourages an overextension of your back. In fact, there are multiple ways to perform back extensions, all correct, and with slight variations in technique that shift the emphasis to different muscles.

To emphasize your lower back and work your spinal erectors dynamically, you encourage a slight overextension of your lower back at the top of the movement. For emphasis on your hamstrings, you push your hips back as you lower and engage through them. And for your glutes, you tuck your chin, flex a little through your thoracic spine to flatten your lumbar curve, and drive your hips into the pad.

If you want to emphasize one muscle over another, then you have options. Otherwise, here's the technique you should use for a more even emphasis and to strengthen your entire posterior chain.

Setup

- Adjust the back extension bench so you can stand on the foot plate with your hip crease level with the top of the pad.
- Hold a weight to your chest if you require extra load.

Performance

1. Initiate the hip hinge by pushing your hips back and hinging over the hip pad.
2. The weight should be through your heels, your knees should be straight but not overly extended, and your back and neck should remain neutral.

3. Lower as far as you can without rounding your spine to complete the movement. You should feel a stretch in your hamstrings.

4. To come up, pinch your glutes together and press your hips into the hip pad.

5. Rise up to the top, but do not overextend your back.

6. Squeeze your glutes, hamstrings, and lower back hard at the top.

7. Inhale as you lower, and exhale as you rise. Engage your core throughout.

Variations

- If you don't have a back extension bench, then try performing back extensions on a stability ball with your feet against a wall.

- Alternatively, you can lie face-down on the floor with your hands behind your head. Lift your chest and legs off the floor while keeping your thighs down. These are sometimes referred to as dorsal raises and are a good no-equipment alternative to back extensions.

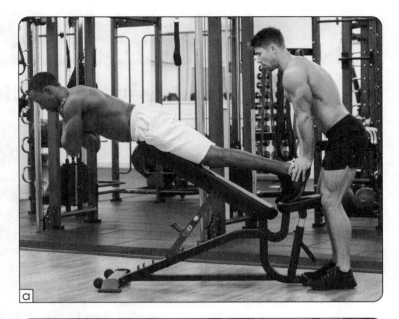

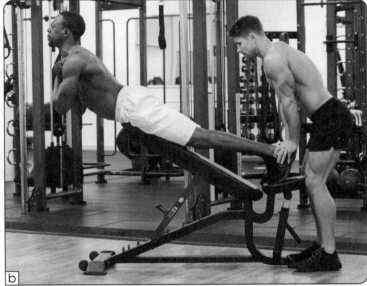

4
CHINESE REVERSE PLANK

Level: Intermediate

You've heard of front and side planks, but how about Chinese reverse planks? While front planks work everything on the front of your body, reverse planks work everything on your backside. When we talk about achieving an optimal balance in strength between muscles, it makes sense that you work everything you can't see just as hard as what you see in the mirror. Exercises like this help you with that.

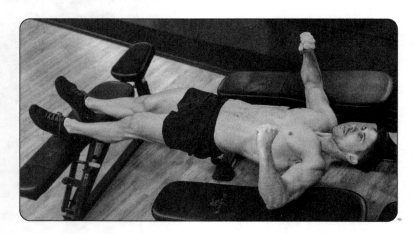

The Chinese reverse plank is an isometric exercise that strengthens your entire posterior chain. Here, that's everything from between your shoulder blades all the way down to your lower legs. Training these muscles will do wonders for your posture as well as provide an excellent way to strengthen and activate a lot of muscles around your backside without the need for much weight.

If you like a challenge, then you're in for one here. Being able to hold a strict Chinese reverse plank for 30 seconds or more is a good standard to accomplish. Any less and you have your work cut out for you. If you're just showing off, then why not try upping the challenge with a weight across your hips, too. This will give your posterior chain the workout it needs.

Setup

- You need three benches, boxes, or chairs of equal height.
- Place two benches approximately shoulder-width apart.
- Place the third bench for your feet to rest on.

Performance

1. Begin by resting your elbows on the two benches near your shoulders.
2. Rest your feet on the bench near your feet.
3. Bend your elbows to 90 degrees, and clench your fists and point them toward the ceiling.
4. Drive your elbows and heels down into the benches to lift yourself.
5. With knees and hips straight, squeeze your hamstrings, glutes, and abs to hold at the top.
6. Keep your elbows pulled down and shoulder blades pinched together.
7. Hold in this position and fight to keep your hips and back from dropping.

Variations

- To make this easier, bring the benches in closer.
- To make this harder, move the benches farther apart or place weight across your hips.
- You can also do these with your feet on the floor and your hips held in a bridged position.

5
CLAM RAISE

Level: Intermediate

Clam raises train your glutes through hip abduction and external rotation. Unlike many similar exercises, clam raises are a good choice for strengthening your glutes because of the limited load through your hip flexors. These muscles tend to be overactive and overpowering, especially if you're doing a lot of abdominal training.

Clam raises are also a great exercise for taking you into the frontal plane. Frontal plane exercises involve moving sideways; most exercises use forward or backward movements.

Being strong in all planes of motion is important, and so is strengthening your glutes. These exercises are best performed as part of a warm-up at the beginning of your workout or near the end for a burning finisher.

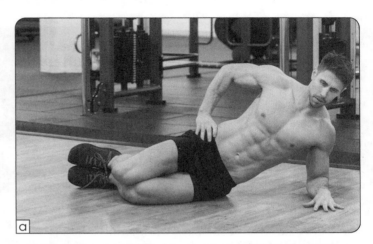

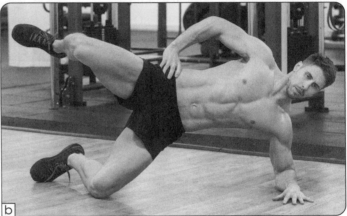

Setup

- Lie on your side on a mat (optional).
- Use foam pads for your elbows and knees if you need extra comfort.
- Bend your knees and hips approximately 90 degrees to start, although you can adjust this depending on how it feels.

Performance

1. Stay on your side as much as you can throughout the movement. This will emphasize hip abduction and external rotation while limiting hip flexor recruitment.
2. Drive your top knee up toward the ceiling and bottom knee down into the floor or foam pad.
3. Open your knees and feet like a clam shell.
4. Raise your bottom hip off the floor at the same time.
5. Focus on squeezing the side area of your glutes. Resting one hand on your top side to feel your glutes engage will help with this.
6. Return your hip to the start position, bringing your knees and feet back toward each other.
7. Complete all of your repetitions on one side before switching to the other.

Variations

- Use a resistance band around your knees as a progression.
- Perform a basic clam as an easier option. Here you'll keep your hips down and feet together throughout. Your knees will still part like a clam.

6
COPENHAGEN HIP ADDUCTION

Level: Intermediate

Training glutes is all the rage for both performance and injury prevention. But the muscles on the other side of your hips are just as important. Despite this, they are often neglected and rarely trained. To achieve optimal muscle balance around your hips, you need to train your adductors frequently. These muscles of the inner thigh include the adductor magnus, adductor longus, adductor brevis, obturator externus, and gracilis.

Copenhagen hip adductions are just one exercise you can use to hit this important group of muscles, and they are relatively scalable for all strength levels. Use Copenhagen hip adductors to improve the strength and resilience of your entire lower body, prevent injury, and carve out strong inner thighs.

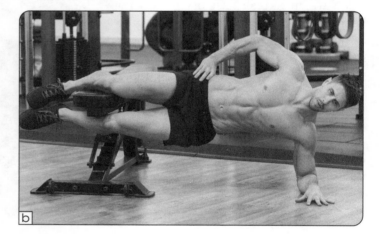

Setup

- For a beginner's version of the Copenhagen hip adduction, begin in a side-lying position with your knee on the bench.
- Your bottom leg is under the bench or just level with the top of the bench, depending on the style of bench you're using.
- Stack your bottom elbow under your shoulder and press it into the floor.
- Use a foam pad for your elbow if needed.

Performance

1. Activating your adductor (inner thigh) muscles, begin to press your top knee into the bench.
2. Keeping your elbow on the floor, your hip will rise to put you into a side bridge position.
3. Your body should be one rigid line at the top of the movement as your legs come together.
4. Lower back to the start.
5. Take one to two seconds to rise and two seconds to lower.
6. Use the breathing technique that is most comfortable for you.

Variations

- For a more advanced progression, make contact with the bench farther down your leg.
- Placing your top foot on the bench makes this exercise the most challenging.
- Use either dynamic repetitions with a controlled tempo, or hold the top position isometrically for time.

The Programs

Part III brings you nine workout programs for all fitness levels that you can do anywhere. From body-weight programs requiring no equipment to home gym and gym-based programs with maximum flexibility, this section has the program that is right for you.

Chapter 12 walks you through essential warm-up options and three body-weight ab workout programs with beginner, intermediate, and advanced options. You'll see some of the best exercises from part II put into action and formulated into a plan that actually works. Using just your own body weight, you'll be able to get in an effective ab workout that leaves no stone unturned. Indeed, with no equipment, you *can* build six-pack abs and an impressive physique.

Chapter 13 offers three workout programs well suited to most average-equipped home gyms. With the rising popularity of working out in backyard and garage gyms, the programs in this chapter give you the best training experience no matter where that might be. With access to dumbbells, kettlebells, and resistance bands, there'll be no holding you back from the exercise options you have available or the results that you can achieve. Some creativity might be needed, but this only adds to the enjoyment of working out from home.

In chapter 14, you'll see what represents the perfect workouts you need to get the fastest results. Gym-based ab workout programs give you the most flexibility in your training plan, and you won't be held back by a lack of specialist equipment or weights. These workouts can be as challenging as you choose to make them and empowering for the complete beginner. There is a plan for you no matter what level you're starting from.

Finally, whether you want to use one of the done-for-you programs or develop your own using the exercises in part II, chapter 15 will show you how to customize your training for unparalleled results. This chapter answers important questions, such as these:

- Is training consistency more important than variation?
- How do you work around injuries?

Part III has something for everyone and is a source of information and inspiration you can revisit time and again.

Body-Weight Ab Workout Programs

Y ou don't need heavy weights or fancy equipment to get in a great workout. By using smart training strategies, your own body can become your gym. This chapter outlines beginner, intermediate, and advanced body-weight workout programs that require no equipment. You might choose one of these programs because you don't have gym access, you're traveling, or you enjoy mastering the ability to use your own body. These exercises are highly effective and can get you closer to your goal of attaining ultimate abs without spending a cent, or for very little cost on equipment you likely already have lying about.

Body-weight programs can reap great results. But you still need to abide by the same training principles that dictate how your body adapts and responds to workouts that were discussed in chapter 1. Performing the same basic front plank or hundreds of basic crunches for months on end will do little to build your abs. Progressive overload needs to take place, and your abdominals need to be challenged in order to get stronger and look better over time.

The body-weight programs in this chapter include beginner (table 12.2), intermediate (table 12.3), and advanced (table 12.4) workout options. Select the program that best reflects your current abilities and aim to perform the workout two or three times each week. This could be your entire training plan if that's all you have time for. Or, for the best results, combine these workouts with a training plan that takes the rest of your body into account, too. For example, you might perform one of this chapter's routines two or three times each week in conjunction with upper- and lower-body workouts other days of the week. If you prefer longer workouts, then you could also use these exercises as add-ons at the end of your current workout routines. For example, do these at the end of a leg workout. You have plenty of options, but the best one is always the one you are most likely to stick to consistently. You should start to see some progress after just a few weeks of using these workout programs. You may also wish to use these workout programs as a basis from which to customize your own workouts, and use what you'll learn in chapter 15 for a more precise training approach.

FOUR-PHASE WARM-UP
FOR ULTIMATE AB WORKOUTS

Just because it's an ab workout doesn't mean you can skip the warm-up. Doing the wrong warm-up (or worse, doing nothing), will lead to a bad workout. That means a workout with less energy, diminished performance, and an increased likelihood of injury. On the other hand, a good warm-up will accomplish the following:

- Unlock hidden muscle strength and power.
- Wake-up dormant muscles.
- Enhance blood flow and nutrient delivery to active muscles.
- Improve oxygen delivery to working muscles.
- Improve reaction times.
- Increase muscle length and range of motion in joints.
- Optimize joint positioning, and correct poor exercise technique.
- Reduce injury potential.
- Increase your ability to run, jump, and throw, faster, higher, and farther.

There is no downside to warming up and a lot to be gained from it. While some rehabilitation specialists suggest foam rolling or isolated mobilization-based warm-ups, others suggest just a 10-minute stroll on any piece of cardio equipment. While there are merits to these techniques, there are better options that check all of the right boxes and prime you better so you're ready for your workouts.

Use the acronym SMAP to perform the ultimate ab warm-up routine. SMAP stands for self-massage, mobilize, activate, and prime. Conducting each step in that order will prepare your body for effective workouts, prevent and even rehabilitate common injuries, and have you breaking personal records.

Phase 1: Self-Massage

Self-massage, sometimes called self-myofascial-release (SMR) technique, is an inhibitory technique that decreases overactivity of the muscular and nervous systems. By using either a foam roller or massage balls of different densities, you can target and apply pressure to tight and overused muscles and painful trigger points. It's frequently referred to as the poor person's massage because it's accessible to anyone and relatively inexpensive.

Self-massage is a highly effective tool for improving the quality of your muscle and connective tissues, increasing blood flow and tissue length, and potentially reducing muscle soreness from previous training sessions. It's no replacement for a professional massage or treatment, but self-massage is practical and can be done almost anywhere.

So often are we focused on the quantity (size and shape) of our muscles that the quality of those tissues is neglected. It's not within the scope of this book to go over specific self-massage exercises, and there are plenty of dedicated resources elsewhere. But you should aim for one to two minutes of self-massage over any areas that are typically overused, are possibly tight, or have painful hot spots or trigger points. Start with a low-density foam roller or large ball, and progress to a higher-density foam roller or massage ball.

Phase 2: Mobilize

The goals of this phase are to restore function to your joints and tissues and reeducate your body to be able to achieve key body positions involved in your workouts—for example, being able to easily get into a half-kneeling position while maintaining optimal body position and stability.

If you're physically unable to get into certain positions and maintain stability, then you need to address the mobility restriction. The best way to complete and customize this approach is to take a test-and-retest approach: Try a half-kneeling position (or other movement of choice), see how it feels, take note of what areas might feel tight or restricted, and then work on mobilizing those areas with specific dynamic stretching exercises. I have specified *dynamic* because that is the only way you should move before your workouts. There are a variety of books and online resources that can give you plenty of options for dynamic stretches. Save your static stretches for afterward if you choose to do them.

After you've completed the dynamic stretches, go back to the original movement. If it has improved, then you know you've been doing the right things. If it hasn't, then you need to go back to the drawing board or spend longer doing them. Keep mobilizing until you feel as though you've made a change to the tight tissues and structures—30 seconds to two minutes should be spent on each exercise. Taking this test-and-retest approach beats doing a bunch of random dynamic stretches any day of the week because you're doing more of what you need and spending less time on what you don't. General areas that often require a little more attention include the big toe, ankle, hamstrings, hip flexors, hips, thoracic spine, shoulders, and wrists.

Phase 3: Activate

The aim of this phase is to activate key muscle groups using low-load exercises that build muscle awareness. This type of exercise is typically used to restore fundamental movement patterns by increasing joint stability and motor control. For the purpose of building your abs, these will increase your awareness of your abs and core so you can target them even better. These low-intensity exercises as part of your warm-up reeducate the deep core stabilizers that typically lie dormant, encouraging them to work more efficiently and priming your nervous system for the workout to follow.

In terms of targeting specific muscle groups or movements, the inclusion of activating exercises will depend on your own needs and weaknesses. Exercises in this category often include those traditionally associated with rehabilitation, such as miniband routines, gluteal activation exercises, light rotator cuff exercises, and low-load core and pelvic floor exercises. Some of these have been included at the start of the programs in chapters 12 through 14; for example, dead bugs and bird dogs. These exercises should not be exhausting and should focus on creating a mind–muscle connection with your abs and core while building body awareness.

Phase 4: Prime

This final phase of your warm-up is optional, but will instantly increase your performance and get your body ready for the best workout possible. It is optional because usually it is reserved for workouts that focus on movement performance after you've developed a basic level of strength in your abs. If you have the time to do them, this phase of your warm-up will enhance your overall results.

Workout performance relies on the existence of both fatigue and postactivation potentiation (PAP). PAP can be seen as the opposite of fatigue, and while one will diminish workout performance, the other will enhance it. More PAP and less fatigue will leave your body in a more primed and ready state and better able to burn body fat. This is great news for both setting your workout personal bests and revealing your abs!

Different types of exercises work to prime your body. For practical purposes, power-based body-weight and resistance band exercises work best. For your whole body, these can include vertical jumps, plyometric push-ups, and even jumping jacks. Exercises for core and abs include chops, rotations, and punches performed explosively with a resistance band. Complete one to three sets of five to seven repetitions of the priming exercise at the end of your four-phase warm-up for the best results (table 12.1).

Table 12.1 Four-Phase Ultimate Ab Warm-Up for a Core and Ab-Focused Workout

Phase	Goal	Exercise focus	Time spent on each phase
1: Self-massage	Loosen tight muscles and areas of the body through nonaggressive soft-tissue techniques	Full body, particularly back and hip flexors	3-5 min
2: Mobilize	Improve joint and tissue mobility using dynamic exercises with swinging or gliding motions	Full body, particularly shoulders, thoracic spine, hips, and ankles	3-5 min
3: Activate	Activate dormant or inactive muscles to improve awareness and coordination	Low-level core exercises, such as dead bugs, bird dogs, and leg lowering; breathing drills	Pick one exercise
4: Prime	Increase strength, power, and performance	Explosive core power exercises such as band chops, rotations, and punches	Pick one exercise

BEGINNER BODY-WEIGHT WORKOUT PROGRAM

If you're coming back to training after time off or are starting from the beginning to build good habits and a foundation, the beginner body-weight program is the best place to start. Table 12.2 lists the best exercises to work your core and abdominals, placing you in perfect positions to improve technique and muscle awareness. This program offers very low risk and a high reward if you focus on performing each exercise as it is described in part II (chapters 7 through 11). Complete each workout two or three times each week for three weeks. After three weeks, then you should move on to the intermediate program (table 12.3) or refer to chapter 15 for tips on customizing. You'll require no equipment and a maximum of 40 minutes, so there really are no excuses to not get after it!

Table 12.2   Beginner Body-Weight Workout Program

	Classification	Page	Week 1	Week 2	Week 3	Make it easier	Make it harder
1. Basic side plank	Foundational	162	2 × 20 seconds e/s Rest 30 seconds between sets.	2 × 30 seconds e/s Rest 30 seconds between sets.	2 × 40 seconds e/s Rest 30 seconds between sets.	Perform on knees.	Add a weight plate or dumbbell on your hips.
2. Basic front plank	Foundational	157	3 × 20 seconds e/s Rest 30 seconds between sets.	3 × 30 seconds e/s Rest 30 seconds between sets.	3 × 40 seconds e/s Rest 30 seconds between sets.	Perform on knees.	Try a long-lever plank.
3. Body-weight Russian twist	Foundational	134	2 × 16-20 alt. Rest 45 seconds between sets.	2 × 24-30 alt. Rest 45 seconds between sets.	2 × 30-40 alt. Rest 45 seconds between sets.	Place feet on the floor for more stability.	Use a small plate, dumbbell, or kettlebell in your hands, as long as quality is maintained.
4. Ab mat crunch (use a rolled-up towel for lower back)	Foundational	91	3 × 8-11* Rest 45 seconds between sets.	3 × 12-14* Rest 45 seconds between sets.	2 × 15-18* Rest 45 seconds between sets.	Perform without the 1- to 2-second pause.	Perform with arms overhead.
5. Basic reverse crunch	Foundational	106	2 × 12-14 Rest 45 seconds between sets.	2 × 15-20 Rest 45 seconds between sets.	2 × 21-30 Rest 45 seconds between sets.	Reduce range of motion.	Lower in 3-4 seconds.

e/s = each side
alt. = alternating reps on each side
* = Add a one- to two-second pause in the top portion of the exercise.

INTERMEDIATE BODY-WEIGHT WORKOUT PROGRAM

The intermediate body-weight workout program (see table 12.3) is a progression of the beginner program. Although it is recommended that you start with the beginner training program to develop a foundation and master perfect technique, you may use the intermediate program right away if you feel it is more suitable to your current level. That is, if you can perform the exercises listed with perfect technique and execution and with a good internal focus on feeling your abdominals contracting with every repetition, you can start with the intermediate program. The beginner and intermediate exercises might look basic to you, but they put you in ideal and uncomplicated positions that allow you to maximize tension in the areas you're targeting. If you don't feel these exercises in your abs, then you're not doing them right and may need to use a beginner program for a while. Perform these workouts two or three times each week alongside your full-body training program for the best overall results. The exercises are made progressively harder over three weeks; after that you might want to try the advanced program (table 12.4) or make up your own program (see chapter 15 on how to customize plans).

Table 12.3 Intermediate Body-Weight Workout Program

	Classification	Page	Week 1	Week 2	Week 3	Make it easier	Make it harder
1. Long-lever plank	Advanced	158	4 × 10 seconds Rest 45 seconds between sets.	3 × 20 seconds Rest 45 seconds between sets.	3 × 25-30 seconds Rest 45 seconds between sets.	Shorten the distance between the elbows and feet.	Move feet and elbows farther apart.
2. Hand walkout	Intermediate	164	3 × 5-7 Rest 60 seconds between sets.	3 × 8-10 Rest 60 seconds between sets.	3 × 8-10* Rest 60 seconds between sets.	Walk hands over a shorter distance.	Walk out farther. Wear a weighted vest.
3. Leg raise	Intermediate	107	3 × 8-12 Rest 45 seconds between sets.	3 × 15 Rest 45 seconds between sets.	3 × 16-20 Rest 45 seconds between sets.	Perform with a slight knee bend.	Lower in 3-4 seconds.
4. Body-weight oblique crunch	Foundational	128	2 × 12-15 e/s Rest 60 seconds between sets.	2 × 15-20 e/s Rest 60 seconds between sets.	2 × 12-20 e/s Rest 60 seconds between sets.	Break repetitions into chunks rather than doing all 12-20 at once.	Focus on adding resistance when possible.
5. Dead bug crunch	Intermediate	93	2 × 12-16 alt. Rest 60 seconds between sets.	2 × 18-20 alt. Rest 60 seconds between sets.	2 × 18-20 alt. Rest 60 seconds between sets.	Break repetitions into chunks rather than doing all 12-20 at once.	Use a small resistance in each hand to increase difficulty.

e/s = each side

alt. = alternating reps on each side

* = Add a one- to two-second pause in the bottom portion of the exercise.

ADVANCED BODY-WEIGHT WORKOUT PROGRAM

The advanced body-weight workout program (table 12.4) should be used only if you have already built your core and abdominals beyond a beginner level and can use good technique and execution. This level is for you if you know how to make your abdominals work hard using the simplest exercises, have exceptional awareness of your muscles contracting, and you're in need of more challenging exercises to take your abs up a level. With eccentric one-arm push-ups and slider body saws to start, you'll work hard from the get-go. Use the advanced workout program two or three times each week for three weeks. After three weeks, you can begin layering in new exercises. See chapter 15 for more details.

Table 12.4   Advanced Body-Weight Workout Program

	Classification	Page	Week 1	Week 2	Week 3	Make it easier	Make it harder
1. Eccentric one-arm push-up	Advanced	180	2 × 4-5 e/s Rest 45 seconds between sets.	2 × 5-6 e/s Rest 45 seconds between sets.	2 × 7-10 e/s Rest 45 seconds between sets.	Perform with hands elevated on a box or bench.	Bring feet in narrower to increase the core challenge.
2. Slider body saw (use paper plates or socks)	Advanced	177	3 × 5-7 Rest 60 seconds between sets.	3 × 8-10 Rest 60 seconds between sets.	3 × 11-15 Rest 60 seconds between sets.	Limit the distance you slide back.	Add pauses at the end, or use slower reps.
3. Hamstring-activated sit-up	Advanced	80	3 × 5-7 Rest 60 seconds between sets.	3 × 8-10 Rest 60 seconds between sets.	2 × 11-15 Rest 60 seconds between sets.	Start from the top. Only lower partially.	Reach arms overhead on the way down.
4. Seated rack toes to bar (use chair or table)	Hardcore	122	2 × 12-15 Rest 45 seconds between sets.	2 × 12-15 Rest 45 seconds between sets.	2 × 12-15 Rest 45 seconds between sets.	Swap the pike for a knee tuck.	Slow repetition speed.
5. Side plank lift	Intermediate	129	2 × 15-20 e/s Rest 45 seconds between sets.	2 × 15-20 e/s Rest 45 seconds between sets.	2 × 15-20 e/s Rest 45 seconds between sets.	Reduce range of motion.	Place a plate or dumbbell on your hips.

e/s = each side

Home Gym Ab Workout Programs

This chapter offers workouts specifically designed for working out at home or in a garage gym environment. They require a limited amount of equipment, which also means using more creative lifting techniques to increase the intensity.

Each of the beginner (table 13.1), intermediate (table 13.2), and advanced (table 13.3) programs are intended to be performed two or three times per week to get the best results. For example, complete the exercises listed in the week 1 workout two or three times that week.

Choose the program that best represents your current abilities and that you can perform consistently for three weeks before moving on to another. After three weeks, you may try one of the more advanced programs, or you can use the information in chapter 15 to build your own.

When performing each workout, remember everything this book has taught you about exercise technique. Next to each exercise is the page number where you can find key coaching points and tips. Always refer to these to get the most out of each exercise and workout. And, above all, enjoy the journey.

BEGINNER HOME WORKOUT PROGRAM

The following home workout program is intended for beginners (table 13.1) or people who want to build a solid abdominal and core foundation before moving on to a more advanced program. Complete each workout a maximum of three times each week on top of your regular strength training routine or in place of your usual workouts. Depending on the program, you'll require just a small amount of equipment, most of which you may already have, or can be purchased for very little cost.

Table 13.1 Beginner Home-Based Workout Program

	Classification	Page	Week 1	Week 2	Week 3	Make it easier	Make it harder
1. Basic bird dog	Foundational	191	2 × 8-10 e/s Rest 30 seconds between sets.	2 × 10-12 e/s Rest 30 seconds between sets.	2 × 12-15 e/s Rest 30 seconds between sets.	Return to the floor after each rep.	Load with a resistance band or small weight.
2. Basic dead bug	Foundational	186	2 × 12-14 alt. Rest 30 seconds between sets.	2 × 16-18 alt. Rest 30 seconds between sets.	2 × 20-24 alt. Rest 30 seconds between sets.	Practice holding the position statically.	Perform with straighter legs.
3. Stir the pot	Intermediate	159	3 × 10-20 seconds Rest 45 seconds between sets.	3 × 15-25 seconds Rest 45 seconds between sets.	3 × 20-30 seconds Rest 45 seconds between sets.	Perform on your knees.	Imagine stirring a bigger pot with a wider arm movement.
4. Body-weight Russian twist	Foundational	134	2 × 16-20 alt. Rest 45 seconds between sets.	2 × 24-30 alt. Rest 45 seconds between sets.	2 × 30-40 alt. Rest 45 seconds between sets.	Place feet on the floor for more stability.	Use a small plate, dumbbell, or kettlebell if quality can be maintained.
5. Stability ball crunch	Intermediate	78	2 × 8-11* Rest 45 seconds between sets.	2 × 12-14* Rest 45 seconds between sets.	2 × 15-18* Rest 45 seconds between sets.	Perform without the 1- to 2-second pause.	Take 4 seconds to lower on each rep.
6. Basic reverse crunch	Foundational	106	2 × 12-14 Rest 45 seconds between sets.	2 × 15-20 Rest 45 seconds between sets.	2 × 15-20* Rest 45 seconds between sets.	Lift off the floor only as far as you can. Increase over time.	Perform with knees slightly straighter.

e/s = each side
alt. = alternating reps on each side
* = Add a one- to two-second pause in the top portion of the exercise.

INTERMEDIATE HOME WORKOUT PROGRAM

The intermediate home workout program (table 13.2) is designed to work if you have already built a solid foundation. You will have experience in using simple exercises and will have focused on executing each repetition perfectly. Compared to the beginner program, this program uses higher exercise complexity and more resistance. Greater resistance can be in the form of external weight or changing lever arm length while using your own body weight. Complete each workout a maximum of three times each week on top of your regular strength training routine or in place of your usual workouts. You'll require an abdominal wheel, a kettlebell, and a stability ball for each workout.

Table 13.2 Intermediate Home-Based Workout Program

	Classification	Page	Week 1	Week 2	Week 3	Make it easier	Make it harder
1. Bear shoulder tap	Intermediate	169	2 × 20 seconds Rest 30 seconds between sets.	2 × 30 seconds Rest 30 seconds between sets.	2 × 40 seconds Rest 30 seconds between sets.	Start with hips in a higher position or in a wider stance.	Make the space between feet and hands narrower.
2. Ab wheel rollout with flexion	Intermediate	100	3 × 8-10 Rest 60 seconds between sets.	3 × 12-15 Rest 60 seconds between sets.	3 × 12-15* Rest 60 seconds between sets.	Set up in front of a wall to limit range of motion with the wheel.	Lower with a 4-second tempo.
3. Kettlebell windmill	Advanced	144	2 × 8-10 e/s Rest 60 seconds between sets.	2 × 12-15 e/s Rest 60 seconds between sets.	2 × 12-15 e/s Rest 60 seconds between sets.	Reduce range of motion by coming only half-way down.	Increase weight.
4. Kettlebell Russian twist	Intermediate	135	2 × 16-20 alt. Rest 45 seconds between sets.	2 × 16-20 alt. Rest 45 seconds between sets.	2 × 16-20 alt. Rest 45 seconds between sets.	Place feet on the floor for more stability.	Increase weight.
5. Hamstring-activated stability ball crunch	Advanced	81	2 × 10-12 Rest 60 seconds between sets.	2 × 12-15 Rest 60 seconds between sets.	2 × 12-15** Rest 60 seconds between sets.	Do without hamstring activation.	Hold a small weight overhead.
6. Banded lying leg raise	Intermediate	119	2 × 12-15 Rest 60 seconds between sets.	2 × 12-15 Rest 60 seconds between sets.	2 × 12-15 Rest 60 seconds between sets.	Perform with bent knees.	Hold a medicine ball between the feet.

e/s = each side

alt. = alternating reps on each side

* = Add a one- to two-second pause in the bottom portion of the exercise.

** = Add a one- to two-second pause in the top portion of the exercise.

ADVANCED HOME WORKOUT PROGRAM

The advanced home workout program (table 13.3) is intended only if you already have a lot of experience using abdominal exercises. Exercises included in this program produce some of the greatest levels of abdominal muscle activation and are of the highest complexity. If you've mastered the beginner and intermediate programs while maintaining great technique and abdominal tension throughout, then use this advanced program to take your abs to the next level. Complete each workout two or three times each week, allowing adequate recovery between each. You'll require a resistance band, core sliders, a stability ball, and a light dumbbell for each workout.

Table 13.3 Advanced Home-Based Workout Program

	Classification	Page	Week 1	Week 2	Week 3	Make it easier	Make it harder
1. Dead bug Pallof press (with band)	Intermediate	189	2 × 16-20 alt. Rest 45 seconds between sets.	2 × 16-20 alt. Rest 45 seconds between sets.	2 × 16-20 alt. Rest 45 seconds between sets.	Decrease band resistance.	Perform with straight knees.
2. Slider body saw	Advanced	177	3 × 6-8 Rest 60 seconds between sets.	3 × 10-12 Rest 60 seconds between sets.	3 × 12-15 Rest 60 seconds between sets.	Limit how far you slide back.	Add a pause on every repetition.
3. Band rotation	Foundational	131	2 × 12-15 e/s Rest 45 seconds between sets.	2 × 12-15 e/s Rest 45 seconds between sets.	2 × 12-15 e/s Rest 45 seconds between sets.	Use a lighter band.	Use a heavier band.
4. Medicine ball walkout	Advanced	173	2 × 5-7 Rest 45 seconds between sets.	2 × 8-10 Rest 45 seconds between sets.	2 × 8-10 Rest 45 seconds between sets.	Reduce the distance you walk out.	Hold for 2 seconds at the bottom of each rep.
5. Sicilian crunch	Advanced	96	2 × 5-7* Rest 60-90 seconds between sets.	2 × 8-10* Rest 60-90 seconds between sets.	2 × 8-10* Rest 60-90 seconds between sets.	Use only body weight.	Increase dumbbell weight.
6. Seated rack toes to bar (if no rack is available, hold on to a table)	Hardcore	122	2 × max reps Rest 45 seconds between sets.	2 × max reps Rest 45 seconds between sets.	2 × max reps Rest 45 seconds between sets.	Use bent knees instead of straight.	Focus on beating max reps attained in previous workout.

e/s = each side

* = Take four seconds to perform the lowering (eccentric) portion of the movement.

Gym-Based Ab Workout Programs

For many people, the gym provides the best environment for making rapid changes in body composition. It provides the ideal environment and range of tools needed to achieve the fastest changes in physique. Chapter 1 discussed the principles behind abdominal training and that you need to build your abs like you would any other muscle. You need to subject your abdominals to hypertrophy training, and a gym gives you the exercise and loading options you need to accomplish this.

In the gym-based programs in this chapter, you'll find beginner (table 14.1), intermediate (table 14.2), and advanced (table 14.3) workout options. These workouts leave no stone unturned for giving you the best exercises to build ultimate abs. Each gym-based program is made up of a mix of exercises that require you to use different pieces of equipment, including cables, free weights, and a landmine. From start to finish, each workout will take you through a full spectrum of exercises that target your abs from every direction. And for the best results, you'll combine these with core exercises to get the best of both aesthetics and function.

Select the program that reflects your current level of training. For the best results, you should ideally do these workout programs in conjunction with workouts for the rest of your body—for example upper-, lower- or full-body workouts on other days of the week. Alternatively, you can add these programs to the end of your current workouts. For example, you might train your lower body for half of the workout, and then use one of the following programs to finish. That's your choice according to your time availability and training schedule.

The best time to do these workouts is at the time that works best for you and that you can stick to consistently. Once you see the results, you'll always look forward to the next one. Enjoy the journey!

BEGINNER GYM-BASED WORKOUT PROGRAM

The beginner gym-based workout program (table 14.1) has been designed for beginners and people wanting to build a good foundation before progressing to the intermediate program (table 14.2). Complete this workout two or three times each week for three weeks, ideally with a day's rest between each. This workout begins with low-level core activation exercises because as they say, "you can't fire a cannonball from a canoe." This will help fire up everything and increase your core and abdominal awareness, so you can perform the heavy-hitter core exercises with the force of a cannonball firing off a battleship. This program finishes with isolated abdominal exercises for the perfect workout.

Table 14.1   Beginner Gym-Based Workout Program

	Classification	Page	Week 1	Week 2	Week 3	Make it easier	Make it harder
1. Banded leg lower	Intermediate	190	2 × 12-16 alt. Rest 30 seconds between sets.	2 × 18-20 alt. Rest 30 seconds between sets.	2 × 20-24 alt. Rest 30 seconds between sets.	Perform with knees bent.	Use a higher resistance band.
2. Miyagi plank	Intermediate	160	3 × 20 seconds e/s Rest 45 seconds between sets.	3 × 30 seconds e/s Rest 45 seconds between sets.	3 × 40 seconds e/s Rest 45 seconds between sets.	Perform on the knees.	Support a small weight on your hips or back.
3. Kettlebell Russian twist	Intermediate	135	3 × 20-24 alt. Rest 45 seconds between sets.	3 × 24-30 alt. Rest 45 seconds between sets.	3 × 30-40 alt. Rest 45 seconds between sets.	Go lighter or do body-weight Russian twist.	Use a heavier kettlebell.
4. Stability ball crunch	Intermediate	78	3 × 12 Rest 45 seconds between sets.	3 × 15 Rest 45 seconds between sets.	3 × 20 Rest 45 seconds between sets.	Perform on the floor with just a mat (optional).	Add a 1- to 2-second pause at the top.
5. Basic reverse crunch	Foundational	106	2 × 12 Rest 45 seconds between sets.	2 × 15 Rest 45 seconds between sets.	2 × 20 Rest 45 seconds between sets.	Reduce range of motion.	Lower in 3-4 seconds.

alt. = alternating reps on each side

INTERMEDIATE GYM-BASED WORKOUT PROGRAM

The intermediate gym-based workout program (table 14.2) has been designed for people who have already built an adequate foundation and have mastered the basic technique and execution of the exercises. Now it's time to introduce more complex exercises to your training and perform more loaded direct work for your abdominals. You'll begin your workout with a low-level core activation exercise to get primed and ready before jumping straight into a workout that will hit your core and abs hard from all directions. Complete this workout two or three times each week, ideally with a day's rest between each. After three weeks, you can layer in different exercises to continue your progress (see chapter 15 to customize your own program). Alternatively, if you feel you can maintain the quality of your workouts and want more challenge, you can try the advanced workout program (table 14.3).

Table 14.2 Intermediate Gym-Based Workout Program

	Classification	Page	Week 1	Week 2	Week 3	Make it easier	Make it harder
1. Dead bug crushing medicine ball	Intermediate	187	2 × 10* e/s Rest 45 seconds between sets.	2 × 12* e/s Rest 45 seconds between sets.	2 × 15* e/s Rest 45 seconds between sets.	Perform basic dead bug.	Hold for 3-4 seconds at the top.
2. Cable antichop	Intermediate	167	3 × 12-15 e/s Rest 60 seconds between sets.	3 × 12-15** e/s Rest 60 seconds between sets.	3 × 12-15** e/s Rest 60 seconds between sets.	Use less cable resistance.	Use more cable resistance.
3. Ab wheel rollout with flexion	Intermediate	100	3 × 8-12 Rest 60 seconds between sets.	3 × 12-15 Rest 60 seconds between sets.	3 × 12-15* Rest 60 seconds between sets.	Perform in front of a wall to reduce range of motion.	Wear a weighted vest.
4. Hamstring-activated reverse crunch	Advanced	111	3 × 12-15 Rest 45 seconds between sets.	3 × 12-20 Rest 45 seconds between sets.	3 × 12-20* Rest 45 seconds between sets.	Perform basic reverse crunches or decline reverse crunches.	Slow the downward phase.
5. Kneeling cable crunch	Foundational	85	3 × 12-20 Rest 45 seconds between sets.	3 × 12-20** Rest 45 seconds between sets.	3 × 12-20** Rest 45 seconds between sets.	Reduce cable weight.	Add cable weight.
6. One-arm farmer's carry	Foundational	165	3 × 60-80 yards e/s Rest 120 seconds between sets.	3 × 60-80 yards e/s Rest 90 seconds between sets.	3 × 60-80 yards e/s Rest 60 seconds between sets.	Reduce dumbbell weight.	Increase dumbbell weight.

e/s = each side

alt. = alternating reps on each side

* = Add a one- to two-second pause at the top.

** = Focus on adding weight from the previous week but achieving the same number of reps.

ADVANCED GYM-BASED WORKOUT PROGRAM

The advanced gym-based workout program (table 14.3) contains exercises with the highest complexity and the greatest loading capacity. If you are at the level to do this program, then you'll see fast results from it. Being at the appropriate level means performing the exercises outlined in table 14.3 with perfect form and execution and feeling every repetition work your abs and core to the max. If you're not able to achieve this, then the advanced program is not for you, and you're better off using the intermediate program (table 14.2). In the advanced program, you'll start with a low-level activation exercise to help fire up your nervous system and get everything primed and ready. You'll then work your core from all angles with some big-hitter exercises, followed by a mix of loaded abdominal exercises that capitalize on different training methods. Perform this workout two or three times each week in conjunction with the rest of your training plan for up to three weeks. After three weeks of planned progression, you can begin to layer in different exercises. Use chapter 15 for reference on how to best customize your plan after giving it your all with this one.

Table 14.3 Advanced Gym-Based Workout Program

	Classification	Page	Week 1	Week 2	Week 3	Make it easier	Make it harder
1. Dead bug Pallof press	Intermediate	189	2 × 12 alt. e/s Rest 45 seconds between sets.	2 × 14 alt. e/s Rest 45 seconds between sets.	2 × 16 alt. e/s Rest 45 seconds between sets.	Perform a basic cable Pallof press.	Use ankle weights for additional leg loading.
2. Landmine squat rainbow	Hardcore	194	3 × 12-16 alt. Rest 60 seconds between sets.	3 × 12-16** alt. Rest 60 seconds between sets.	3 × 12-16** alt. Rest 60 seconds between sets.	Perform the regular landmine rainbow.	Add weight.
3. Barbell ab rollout	Advanced	171	3 × 8-12 Rest 60 seconds between sets.	3 × 12-15 Rest 45 seconds between sets.	3 × 12-15* Rest 45 seconds between sets.	Perform in front of a wall to reduce range of motion.	Wear a weighted vest.
4. Garhammer leg raise	Advanced	121	3 × AMGRAP Rest 60 seconds between sets.	3 × AMGRAP Rest 60 seconds between sets.	3 × AMGRAP Rest 60 seconds between sets.	Perform the seated rack toes to bar.	Slow repetition speed.
5. Sicilian crunch	Advanced	96	3 × 10-12 Rest 90 seconds between sets.	3 × 10-12** Rest 90 seconds between sets.	3 × 10-12** Rest 90 seconds between sets.	Perform the hamstring-activated stability ball crunch.	Add weight.
6. Incline plate Russian twist	Intermediate	137	2 × 20-30 alt. Rest 60 seconds between sets.	2 × 20-30** alt. Rest 60 seconds between sets.	2 × 20-30** alt. Rest 60 seconds between sets.	Perform the landmine full- or half-core rotation.	Increase the degree of incline or increase the weight.

e/s = each side

alt. = alternating reps on each side

alt. e/s = alternating legs and on each side

* = Add a one- to two-second pause at the top.

** = Focus on adding weight from the previous week but achieving the same number of reps.

AMGRAP = as many good repetitions as possible

Customizing Your Own Program

By reading this book, you have developed a deeper understanding of exercise selection and programming for ab and core training, which are based on sound scientific principles. You've learned what types of exercises are the best for building your abs. You've also learned about performance- and prevention-based exercises that complement your six-pack training. You've built a database of exercises that could last you a lifetime of training and done-for-you workout programs that keep you from having to do any guesswork. Chapters 12, 13, and 14 outlined a variety of workout programs suitable for all ability levels and equipment availability. This chapter shows you how to take what you've learned and the programs outlined in previous chapters and customize them to your own body.

CUSTOMIZING EXERCISE SELECTION

Any well-structured training program starts with setting clearly defined goals. This is followed by the strategic planning phase and then progression. There should be no training randomness or hopping from one program to another. Instead, training should be purposeful and justified of all of your efforts. A good training program will never have you beating up your body or feeling like your muscles and joints are permanently sore. Training should *stimulate* and not *annihilate* your body. This is how your body adapts and gets better. A massive part of accomplishing this is knowing how to select the right exercises for your anatomy.

At this point, you likely have a better idea than most people do about what the most effective exercises are for training your abs and core. These exercises are based on levels of muscle activation and the ways in which they stimulate your abs to grow. You also have an excellent understanding of what it means to train your core. But you also need to understand that the best exercise for X or Y doesn't always mean it's the best for you.

The previous chapters have given you all the tools you need to get in your best shape ever. But it's also understood that you might get better results using some tools more often than others. You should always look for the right tools (exercises) to fit the program your body needs rather than trying to force the wrong tools to fit. In other words, exercises are general tools, but exercisers are individuals. For example, heavy barbell deadlifts are highly regarded. But as many people eventually find out, performing a straight barbell deadlift from the floor isn't always the best option for them. This can be for many reasons that are outside the scope of this book. However, it's an example of one exercise that is frequently claimed to be beneficial for everyone, yet is not a good choice for many people.

When exercises are selected based on cookie-cutter approaches and universally claimed "best" exercises, then negative things start to happen. Exercises that place your limbs and joints in poor alignment result in unwanted wear and tear and eventual injury. Exercises you use now might not put you in an ideal position to feel that you're working the target muscle, and they may even trigger pain or inflammation. Yet you keep doing these exercises because someone told you they were the best. Thinking you *have* to do certain exercises is often the one thing holding you back from lifelong progress.

You should select exercises based on how they feel when setting up, how they feel when you're performing them (does it work the muscle as intended?), and how you feel in the days afterward. If you've been using one of the programs outlined in chapters 12, 13, or 14, and one of the exercises doesn't feel right, then substitute another. You have my permission to do so! These programs were put together with a general population of beginner, intermediate, and experienced people in mind. I wish I knew more about you and could individualize a program for you, but that's not possible. What is possible, though, is that you pay attention to how each exercise feels and ensure you're doing only the exercises that feel the best. Every exercise in this book was chosen because it's useful and deserves to be in your toolbox. All you need to do is open the toolbox and find something that fits better. Because we've placed exercises into categories according to their movement patterns, finding a good substitute that works the same pattern should be easy.

ACHIEVING CONSISTENCY AND VARIETY AT THE SAME TIME

Consistent workouts are important. Consistently using similar exercises for several weeks is also important so you can get the most out of them. Doing so allows you to track your personal bests and better progress your workouts. Sticking with the same exercises for too long, though, can become monotonous. Not only that, but your progress starts to stall after some time using the same exercises. Repeated use of the same movements can also increase your risk of overuse injuries. Therefore, rotation within your exercise selection is important. This is the layering of exercises mentioned throughout the book.

Exercise layering is one of the best ways to create consistency within your workout programs while introducing variety at the same time. It also factors in that some exercises you do might progress faster than others, so they need to be changed more frequently. Layering within a training program is simply a case of starting with one (consistent) training plan, and then, as you go along, changing up just an exercise or two as you make progress in that plan. This is in contrast to doing a completely different workout every week or changing the whole plan after doing it once.

You can substitute exercises in your program frequently, providing you maintain an element of consistency at the same time. To do this, you might keep your most important exercises (the ones you want to work really hard on improving) in your workout program for an entire month. Repeating these important exercises for three or four weeks will allow time for you to master and get stronger at them but without reaching a plateau. On the other hand, your exercises that are less important can be changed a lot sooner—as often as every workout or two. You can swap out these less important exercises because of the challenge, the urge to experiment, or even if you just get bored easily.

Consistency is important because it allows progression. This is why hopping from one program to another holds so many people back; they don't use an exercise long enough for their body to adapt and progress with it. Variety is an important part of programming psychology though, and it can allow greater progression if exercises are layered in strategically. Variety is also more important for beginners because the more experience you have with a variety of exercises, the more opportunity you will have to learn what feels right and what your body responds to best. This helps you narrow your exercise choices to those that work best.

WORKING AROUND INJURIES

Part II is packed full of exercises that are both safe and highly effective. Although attaining six-pack abs is a clear priority, you also want to do so in a manner that is joint friendly and will maximize your training longevity. This is one of the reasons chapter 10 includes core exercises that attain greater back health and performance. That being said, as was already mentioned, not every exercise will necessarily be a good fit for you. You may be working around old injuries or cranky joints. These are things that exercise can help, but it can also worsen injuries if you're not doing the right things. This is when you need to learn how to modify an exercise to fit you better or try something else to avoid the area completely.

In part II, each exercise is described—what it's good for and how it can be made harder or easier. I hope these descriptions allow you to feel you can experiment with these exercises to get the best workouts for you while avoiding pain and discomfort. I also hope that an understanding of the mechanics of certain exercises sparks creativity. You now have a better idea of how an exercise might be modified to fit you better or work you in a different way. These modifications could be as simple as reducing your range of motion to avoid pain or using a foam pad to raise your back knee higher to avoid hip pain.

Selecting exercises to work around injuries or unwanted pain comes down to this: Select the exercises that allow you to place load through the target area (feeling the muscle working is good pain), while avoiding the unwanted pain (this is bad pain). It really is that simple, and your body in a few years will thank you for it.

CUSTOMIZING TRAINING VOLUME

In chapter 1, we discussed key ab-building principles and how training volume is an extremely important part of programming. We also saw research that indicates the best training volume varies from person to person. This is largely because of genetic and lifestyle factors. For example, while one person might achieve the best results performing 22 sets of an exercise per muscle per week, another person may only require 8. We saw that a general recommendation for volume is to complete 10 to 20 sets of an exercise per muscle group per week. This is a broad range though, and you should experiment to find the training volume that works best for you. It is important to note that often with training volume, less is more—especially as we get older. And the amount you are using now might be too much to stimulate increases in strength and muscle size.

The ab workout programs in chapters 12, 13, and 14 are relatively high on the volume scale. They are specialization programs that are intended to be done for short periods of time. Attempting to keep your ab-focused training volume this high for a long time will likely slow your progress. A better approach is to use a high-volume program like those outlined in chapters 12, 13, and 14 for three to six weeks, then follow up with a lower-volume phase for your abs. For example, perform just 10 sets per week of abdominal training during this period. You could work on other body parts in that time while your abs recover from the previous work and continue to grow. Be willing to experiment with your training volume and what works for you; 10 to 20 sets per week for your abs is a good starting point as a normal training volume for most of the year. Periods of focused training for individual muscle groups can go higher, but not for too long.

WHAT'S NEXT?

You have now taken a complete journey through everything you need to know about building a set of abs and a core you can be proud of: the basic ab-building principles in chapter 1, the anatomy and nuances of different training approaches in chapters 2 through 4, how to assess your progress in chapter 5, a complete toolbox of the best ab and core exercises in chapters 6 through 11, and then the done-for-you workout programs in chapters 12 through 14. The aim of this journey was to give you an education in what it takes to build ultimate abs. We understand that each area discussed is only the tip of the iceberg. You *could* seek more details in each of these areas if you want to. But it's important not to get too stuck in the weeds or allow overthinking to stop you from putting in the actual work. Information without action is indeed useless! This book provides you with everything you need to know and nothing you don't. It's up to you to put in the effort and apply its teachings.

For extra accountability, you can use the hashtag #UltimateAbsBook on Instagram when doing any of the exercises featured in this book. Or tag @humankinetics and @thefitnessmaverick for a chance for it to be shared. You can also keep us updated with your ultimate abs progress if you want to inspire others with your transformation.

Bibliography

Chapter 1

1. Dalton, P.A., and M.J Stokes. 1991. "Acoustic Myography Reflects Force Changes During Dynamic Concentric and Eccentric Contractions of the Human Biceps Brachii Muscle." *European Journal of Applied Physiology* 63: 412-416.

2. Kraemer, R.R., D.B. Hollander, G.V. Reeves, M. Francois, Z.G. Ramadan, Meeker, B. Tryniecki, J.L. et al. 2006. "Similar Hormonal Responses to Concentric and Eccentric Muscle Actions Using Relative Loading." *European Journal of Applied Physiology* 96: 551-557.

3. Schoenfeld, B.J., D.I. Ogborn, A.D. Vigotsky, M.V. Franchi, and J.W. Krieger. 2017. "Hypertrophic Effects of Concentric vs. Eccentric Muscle Actions." *Journal of Strength and Conditioning Research* 31(9): 2599-2608.

4. De Souza-Teixeira, F., and J.A. De Paz. 2012. "Eccentric Resistance Training and Muscle Hypertrophy." *Journal of Sports Medicine and Doping Studies* S1:004.

5. Oranchuk, D.J., A.G. Storey, A.R. Nelson, and J.B. Cronin. 2019. "Scientific Basis for Eccentric Quasi-Isometric Resistance Training." *Journal of Strength and Conditioning Research* 33(10): 2846-2859.

6. Aspe, R.R., and P.A. Swinton. 2014. "Electromyographic and Kinetic Comparison of the Back Squat and Overhead Squat." *Journal of Strength and Conditioning Research* 28(10): 2827-2836.

7. Taber, C.B., A. Vigotsky, G. Nuckols, and C.T. Haun. 2019. "Exercise-Induced Myofibrillar Hypertrophy Is a Contributory Cause of Gains in Muscle Strength." *Sports Medicine* 49: 993-997.

8. Schoenfeld, B.J. 2010. "The Mechanisms of Muscle Hypertrophy and Their Application to Resistance Training." *Journal of Strength and Conditioning Research* 24(10): 2857-2272.

9. Lacerda, L.T., H.C. Martins-Costa, R.C.R. Diniz, F.V. Lima, A.G.P. Andrade, F.D. Tourino, M.G. Bemben, and M.H. Chagas. 2016. "Variations in Repetition Duration and Repetition Numbers Influence Muscular Activation and Blood Lactate Response in Protocols Equalized by Time Under Tension." *Journal of Strength and Conditioning Research* 30(1): 251-258.

10. Häggmark T., and A. Thorstensson. 1979. "Fibre Types in Human Abdominal Muscles." *Acta Physiologica Scandinavica* 107(4): 319-325.

11. Gollnick, P.D., B. Sjödin, J. Karlsson, E. Jansson, and B. Saltin. 1974. "Human Soleus Muscle: A Comparison of Fiber Composition and Enzyme Activities With Other Leg Muscles." *Pflügers Archiv* 348(3) 247-255.

12. Schoenfeld, B.J., D. Ogborn, and J.W. Krieger. 2016. "Dose-Response Relationship Between Weekly Resistance Training Volume and Increases in Muscle Mass: A Systematic Review and Meta-Analysis." *Journal of Sports Sciences* 35(11): 1-10.

13. Scarpelli, M.C., S.R. Nóbrega, N. Santanielo, L.F. Alvarez, G.B. Otoboni, C. Ugrinowitsch, and C.A. Libardi. 2020. "Muscle Hypertrophy Response Is Affected by Previous Resistance Training Volume in Trained Individuals." *Journal of Strength and Conditioning Research*, volume publish ahead of print.

14. Schoenfeld, B.J., and J. Grgic. 2017. "Evidence-Based Guidelines for Resistance Training Volume to Maximize Muscle Hypertrophy." *Strength and Conditioning Journal* 40(4): 1.

15. Grgic, J., B.J. Schoenfeld, T.B. Davies, B. Lazinica, J.W. Krieger, and C. Pedicic. 2018. "Effect of Resistance Training Frequency on Gains in Muscular Strength: A Systematic Review and Meta-Analysis." *Sports Medicine* 48: 1207-1220.

16. Baz-Valle, E., B.J. Schoenfeld, J. Torres-Unda, J. Santos-Concejero, and C. Balsalobre-Fernández. 2019. "The Effects of Exercise Variation in Muscle Thickness, Maximal Strength and Motivation in Resistance Trained Men." *PLoS ONE*, 14(12).

Chapter 2

1. Teyhen, D.S., N.W. Gill, J.L. Whittaker, S.M. Henry, J.A. Hides, and P. Hodges. 2007. "Rehabilitative Ultrasound Imaging of the Abdominal Muscles." *Journal of Orthopaedic and Sports Physical Therapy* 37(8): 450-466.

2. McGill, S.M. 1991. "Electromyographic Activity of the Abdominal and Low Back Musculature During the Generation of Isometric and Dynamic Axial Trunk Torque: Implications for Lumbar Mechanics." *Journal of Orthopaedic Research* 9(1): 91-103.

3. Hamlyn, N., D.G. Behm, and W.B. Young. 2007. "Trunk Muscle Activation During Dynamic Weight-Training Exercises and Isometric Instability Activities." *Journal of Strength and Conditioning Research* 21(4): 1108-1112.

4. Willardson, J., F.E. Fontana, and E. Bressel. 2009. "Effect of Surface Stability on Core Muscle Activity for Dynamic Resistance Exercises." *International Journal of Sports Physiology and Performance* 4(1): 97-109.

5. McGill, S.M., A. McDermott, and C.M. Fenwick. 2009. "Comparison of Different Strongman Events: Trunk Muscle Activation and Lumbar Spine Motion, Load, and Stiffness." *Journal of Strength and Conditioning Research* 23(4): 1148-1161.

6. Duncan, M. 2009. "Muscle Activity of the Upper and Lower Rectus Abdominis During Exercises Performed on and off a stability ball." *Journal of Bodywork and Movement Therapies* 13(4): 364-367.

7. Imai, A., K. Kaneoka, Y. Okubo, I. Shiina, M. Tatsumura, S. Izumi, and H. Shiraki. 2010. "Trunk Muscle Activity During Lumbar Stabilization Exercises on Both a Stable and Unstable Surface." *Journal of Orthopaedic and Sports Physical Therapy* 40(6): 369-375.

8. Atkins, S.J., I. Bentley, D. Brooks, M.P. Burrows, H.T. Hurst, and J.K, Sinclair. 2015. "Electromyographic Response of Global Abdominal Stabilizers in Response to Stable- and Unstable-Base Isometric Exercise." *Journal of Strength and Conditioning Research* 29(6): 1609-1615.

9. Aspe, R.R., and P.A. Swinton. 2014. "Electromyographic and Kinetic Comparison of the Back Squat and Overhead Squat." *Journal of Strength and Conditioning Research* 28(10): 2827-2836.

10. Stenger, E.M. 2013. "Electromyographic Comparison of a Variety of Abdominal Exercises to the Traditional Crunch." Master's thesis. College of Exercise and Sport Science Clinical Exercise Physiology, University of Wisconsin-Lacrosse.

11. McGill, S.M. 2010. "Core Training: Evidence Translating to Better Performance and Injury Prevention." *Strength and Conditioning Journal* 32(3): 33-45.

12. McGill, S.M. 2017. *Ultimate Back Fitness and Performance Sixth Edition*. Champaign, IL: Human Kinetics.

13. Schuler, L., and A. Cosgrove. 2010. *The New Rules of Lifting for Abs: A Myth-Busting Fitness Plan for Men and Women Who Want a Strong Core and a Pain-Free Back*. New York, NY: Avery.

14. Contreras, M.A., and B. Schoenfeld. 2011. "To Crunch or Not to Crunch: An Evidence-Based Examination of Spinal Flexion Exercises, Their Potential Risks, and Their Applicability to Program Design." *Strength and Conditioning Journal* 33(4): 8-18.

15. Videman, T., M. Nurminen, and J.D. Troup. 1990. "Lumbar Spinal Pathology in Cadaveric Material in Relation to History of Back Pain, Occupation, and Physical Loading." *Spine* 15: 728-740.

Chapter 3

1. Juker, D., S. McGill, P. Kropf, and T. Steffen. 1998. "Quantitative Intramuscular Myoelectric Activity of Lumbar Portions Of Psoas and the Abdominal Wall During a Wide Variety of Tasks." *Medicine and Science in Sports and Exercise* 30: 301-310.

2. Sullivan, W., F.A. Gardin, C.R. Bellon, and S. Leigh. 2015. "Effect of Traditional vs. Modified Bent-Knee Sit-Up on Abdominal and Hip Flexor Muscle Electromyographic Activity." *Journal of Strength and Conditioning Research* 29(12): 3472-3479.

3. Larson, D.S., B. Pederson, A. Suedel, and W. Both. 2007. "The Effect of Hamstring Contractions in the Activation of the Abdominal Muscles During a Standard Abdominal Crunch." PhD diss., University of North Dakota.

4. Guimaraes, A.C. , M.A. Vaz, M.I. De Campos, and R. Marantes. 1991. "The Contribution of the Rectus Abdominis and Rectus Femoris in Twelve Selected Abdominal Exercises: An Electromyographic Study." *Journal of Sports Medicine and Physical Fitness* 31: 222-230

5. Moraes, A.C., R.S. Pinto, M.J. Valamatos, M.J. Valamatos, P.L. Pezarat-Correia, A.H. Okano, P.M. Santos, and J.M. Cabri. 2009. "EMG Activation of Abdominal Muscles in the Crunch Exercise Performed With Different External Loads." *Physical Therapy in Sport* 10: 57-62.

6. Sarti, M.A., M. Monfort, M.A. Fuster, and L.A. Villaplana. 1996 "Muscle Activity in Upper and Lower Rectus Abdominus During Abdominal Exercises." *Archives of Physical Medicine and Rehabilitation* 77(12): 1293-1297.

7. Workman, J.C., D. Docherty, K.C. Parfrey, D.G. Behm. 2008. "Influence of Pelvis Position on the Activation of Abdominal and Hip Flexor Muscles. *Journal of Strength and Conditioning Research* 22(5): 1563-1569.

8. Escamilla, R.F., E. Babb, R. DeWitt, P. Jew, P. Kelleher, T. Burnham, J. Busch, K. D'Anna, R. Mowbray, and R.T. Imamura. 2006. "Electromyographic Analysis of Traditional and Nontraditional Abdominal Exercises: Implications for Rehabilitation and Training." *Physical Therapy* 86(5): 656-671.

9. Escamilla, R.F., C. Lewis, and D. Bell. 2010. "Core Muscle Activation During stability ball and Traditional Abdominal Exercises." *Journal of Orthopaedic and Sports Physical Therapy* 40(5): 265-276.

10. Cugliari, G., and G. Boccia. 2017. "Core Muscle Activation in Suspension Training Exercises." *Journal of Human Kinetics* 56(1): 61-71.

11. Stenger, E.M. 2013. "Electromyographic Comparison of a Variety of Abdominal Exercises to the Traditional Crunch." Master's thesis. College of Exercise and Sport Science Clinical Exercise Physiology, University of Wisconsin-Lacrosse.

12. Schoenfeld, B.J., C. Contreras, G. Tiryaki-Sonmez, J.M. Willardson, and F. Fontana. 2014. "An Electromyographic Comparison of a Modified Version of the Plank With a Long Lever and Posterior Tilt Versus the Traditional Plank Exercise." *Sports Biomechanics* 13(3): 296-306.

13. Byrne, J.M., N.S. Bishop, A.M. Caines, K.A. Crane, A.M. Feaver, and G.E.P. Pearcey. 2014. "Effect of Using a Suspension Training System on Muscle Activation During the Performance of a Front Plank Exercise." *Journal of Strength and Conditioning Research* 28(11): 3049-3055.

14. Cortell-Tormo, J.M., M. García-Jaén, I. Chulvi-Medrano, S. Hernández-Sánchez, A.G. Lucas-Cuevas, and J. Tortosa-Martínez. 2017. "Influence of Scapular Position on the Core Musculature Activation in the Prone Plank Exercise." *Journal of Strength and Conditioning Research* 31(8): 2255-2262.

15. Yun, B.G., S.J. Lee, H.J. So, and W.S. Shin. 2017. "Changes in Muscle Activity of the Abdominal Muscles According to Exercise Method and Speed During Dead Bug Exercise." *Physical Therapy Rehabilitation Science* 6(1): 1-6.

16. Santana, J.C., F.J. Vera-Garcia, and S.M. McGill. 2007. "A Kinetic and Electromyographic Comparison of the Standing Cable Press and Bench Press." *Journal of Strength and Conditioning Research* 21(4): 1271-1277.

17. McGill, S.M., A. McDermott, and C.M.J. Fenwick. 2009. Comparison of Different Strongman Events: Trunk Muscle Activation and Lumbar Spine Motion, Load, and Stiffness." *Journal of Strength and Conditioning Research* 23(4): 1148-1161.

18. Calatayud, J., F. Martin, J.C. Colado, J.C. Benítez, M.D. Jakobsen, and L.L. Andersen. 2015. "Muscle Activity During Unilateral vs. Bilateral Battle Rope Exercises." *Journal of Strength and Conditioning Research* 29(10): 2854-2859.

Chapter 4

1. Trexler, E., A. Smith-Ryan, and L. Norton. 2014. "Metabolic Adaptation to Weight Loss: Implications for the Athlete." *Journal of the International Society of Sports Nutrition* 11(7): 1550-2783.

2. Von Loeffelholz, C., and A. Birkenfeld. 2018. "The Role of Non-exercise Activity Thermogenesis in Human Obesity." *Endotext* April 9, 2018.

3. Glickman, N., H.H. Mitchell, E.H. Lambert, and R.W. Keeton. 1948. "The Total Specific Dynamic Action of High-Protein and High-Carbohydrate Diets on Human Subjects: Two Figures." *The Journal of Nutrition* 36(1): 41-57.

4. Mikkola, J., H. Rusko, M. Izquierdo, E.M. Gorostiaga, and K. Häkkinen. 2012. "Neuromuscular and Cardiovascular Adaptations During Concurrent Strength and Endurance Training in Untrained Men." *International Journal of Sports Medicine* 33(9): 702-710.

5. M.R. Rhea, R.L. Hunter, and T.J. Hunter. 2006. "Competition Modeling of American Football: Observational Data and Implications for High School, Collegiate, and Professional Player Conditioning." *Journal of Strength and Conditioning Resources* 20(1): 58-61.

Chapter 5

1. Lee, S.Y., S. Ahn, Y.J. Kim, M.J. Ji, K.M. Kim, S.H. Choi, H.C. Jang, and S. Lim. 2018. "Comparison Between Dual-Energy X-Ray Absorptiometry and Bioelectrical Impedance Analyses for Accuracy in Measuring Whole Body Muscle Mass and Appendicular Skeletal Muscle Mass." *Nutrients* 10(6): 738.

2. Wang, H., S. Hai, L. Cao, J. Zhou, P. Liu, and B.R. Dong. 2016. "Estimation of Prevalence of Sarcopenia by Using a New Bioelectrical Impedance Analysis in Chinese Community-Dwelling Elderly People." *BMC Geriatrics* 16(1): 216.

3. España Romero, V., J.R. Ruiz, F.B. Ortega, E.G. Artero, G. Vicente-Rodríguez, L.A. Moreno, M.J. Castillo, and A. Gutierrez. 2009. "Body Fat Measurement in Elite Sport Climbers: Comparison of Skinfold Thickness Equations With Dual Energy X-Ray Absorptiometry." *Journal of Sports Sciences* 27(5): 469-477.

About the Author

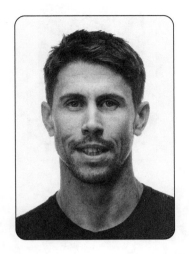

Gareth Sapstead has a master's degree in strength and conditioning science and a bachelor's degree in sports and exercise science, and he holds the NSCA CSCS (Certified Strength and Conditioning Specialist) certification. In the fitness industry since 2005, he has worked with elite soccer players, professional rugby union athletes, and teams across the United Kingdom and Europe as a strength and conditioning specialist. He has also trained Fortune 500 global executives as well as various high-profile clients, physique competitors, and plenty of ordinary people with "dad bods."

Sapstead's name and articles have appeared on some of the world's leading fitness and bodybuilding websites, including T-Nation, Muscle & Strength, *Muscle & Fitness,* and Livestrong, among others. He has self-published three books and coauthored *The Complete Running and Marathon Book* (published by Dorling Kindersley). He's a published researcher in the field of exercise performance and has presented at numerous academic conferences. Sapstead also maintains a popular fitness blog at www.thefitnessmaverick.com.

You read the book—now complete the companion CE exam to earn continuing education credit!

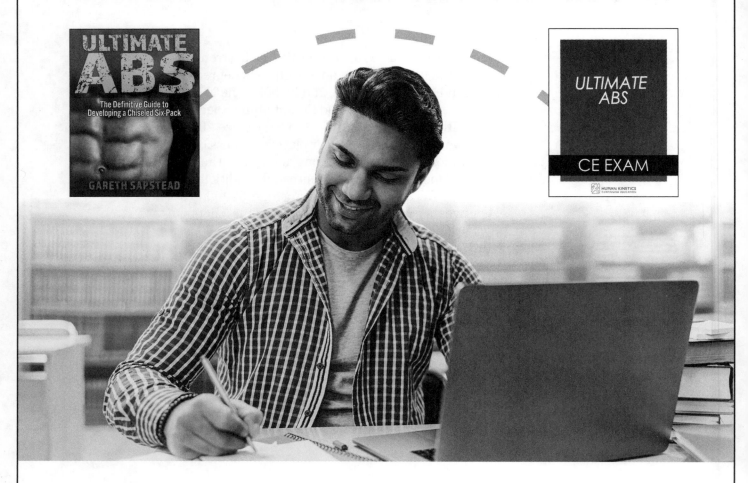

Find and purchase the companion CE exam here:
US.HumanKinetics.com/collections/CE-Exam
Canada.HumanKinetics.com/collections/CE-Exam

50% off the companion CE exam with this code

UA2022

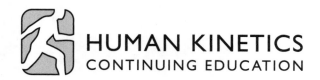

HUMAN KINETICS
CONTINUING EDUCATION